Juliet Richters has worked in sex research and education for over 20 years. She worked on one of Australia's earliest HIV/AIDS prevention research studies, the Condom Project, which included a world first—a study to measure men's erect penises to check appropriate condom sizes. She has lectured and published on health, gender and sexuality and now works for the National Centre in HIV Social Research.

Chris Rissel has worked in all aspects of health promotion research and practice, which has included a focus on sexual health over the last 10 years. He lectures on a variety of technical and advocacy issues and is a prolific writer.

Doing it Down Under

The sexual lives of Australians

Juliet Richters BA, MPH, PhD
Chris Rissel BSc, MPH, PhD

Based on the Australian Study of Health and Relationships, a national representative sample telephone survey of people aged 16 to 59. Principal investigators: Associate Professor Anthony Smith, Dr Chris Rissel, Dr Andrew Grulich and Dr Juliet Richters, with senior research officer Dr Richard de Visser.

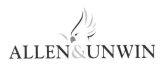

ALLEN&UNWIN

Allen & Unwin
85 Alexander Street
Crows Nest NSW 2065
Australia
Phone: (61 2) 8425 0100
Fax: (61 2) 9906 2218
Email: info@allenandunwin.com
Web: www.allenandunwin.com

National Library of Australia
Cataloguing-in-Publication entry:

Richters, Juliet.
    Doing it Down Under: the sexual lives of Australians.
    Bibliography.
    Includes index.
    ISBN 1 74114 326 8.

    1. Australians – Sexual behaviour. 2. Sexual behaviour surveys –
    Australia. I. Rissel, Chris. II. Title.

306. 70994

Typeset in 10/12pt Bk Hiroshige Book by Midland Typesetters,
Maryborough, Victoria
Printed in Australia by Griffin Press, South Australia

10 9 8 7 6 5 4 3 2 1

contents

acknowledgments

Our first thanks go to our co-researchers on the team for the Australian Study of Health and Relationships, Anthony Smith and Andrew Grulich, and our wonderful research officer Richard de Visser. We are all very grateful to Lorraine Winchester for sorting out the sampling, the Hunter Valley Research Foundation for making the huge and complex questionnaire into a workable computer program, and to the team of immensely professional interviewers. Thanks also to our colleagues and associates around Australia and overseas who advised on the questionnaire and the conduct of the study, all named in the journal articles of the main report (see 'References and further reading').

We are grateful to the editors of the *Australian and New Zealand Journal of Public Health (ANZJPH)* for granting permission to reprint passages that were published in the journal articles reporting the study's main findings. Thanks to Richard de Visser, by then at Birkbeck College in London, and Simon Mamone, research officer at the Australian Research Centre in Sex, Health and Society, for further analyses of the data that were not reported in the original articles, and to Christy Newman for research assistance in Sydney.

Many of our friends, family and colleagues read and commented on drafts of parts or all of the book: thanks to Bernadette Carrigan, Adrian Colman, Randal Colman, Robyn Colman, Jean Edwards, Pol McCann, Christy Newman, Alan Whelan and Trudy Rissel. All errors and confusing sentences that remain are our own responsibility.

preface

These days people are bombarded with advice and information about sex and relationships. Most popular magazines—for both men and women—focus on little else. Headlines scream 'How to give great head', 'Seven ways to amaze her in bed', 'Is your boyfriend cheating on you?', 'Multiple orgasm made easy!' or 'Ten steps to relationship bliss'. Advice columns by doctors and counsellors dispense sexual guidance to readers anxious to know whether their genitals are normal, or how to perform fellatio without gagging, or whether it's true that many people have anal intercourse.

This book, based on survey research, is different from most books about sex that give advice about relationships. We don't start out with any preconceived ideas about what people 'ought' to do sexually. We're not in the business of prescribing sexual morality, or trying to improve marriages or to prevent teenage pregnancy or even HIV infection—though some of the data we present will be useful for those purposes. We simply set out to find out what most Australians do sexually, and what they know and think about sex and sexual health. To do this, we telephoned households nationally to get a sample of Australians aged over sixteen and under sixty and invited them to take part in the study. Nearly twenty thousand people took part, making this the largest sex survey ever done in Australia.

This book was written by us (Chris Rissel and Juliet Richters), but the research work on which is it based was carried out by a team headed by Chris for the pilot study in 1999 and Anthony Smith for the main study in 2000–03. The interviewing was done by the staff of the Hunter Valley Research Foundation using a questionnaire written by the research team. In the book we (the authors) often use the word 'we' to mean the researchers and/or the interviewers, but we do not mean to claim that the survey was all our own work. For more information about how the survey was done, see the appendices.

We have tried to write this book in a simple style to make the information accessible to most people. It is likely to be of particular interest to professionals such as nurses, counsellors, social workers, health educators, school teachers, doctors, sociologists or researchers, but also to everyone who has an interest in the way we live. For those people interested in more statistical and methodological detail, the 'References and further reading' section at the end of the book contains details of the academic articles reporting the survey findings on which each chapter is based. Details of any other research we have drawn on can also be found there, together with suggestions for books and articles of interest to readers seeking further knowledge on each chapter's topic.

For convenience and because it is familiar, we have used the term 'opposite-sex' (as in 'Men report more opposite-sex partners than women do'). However, we do not mean to imply that males and females are sexual opposites. They are more alike than different, and where the sexes do consistently differ, they are not necessarily complementary.

Studying sexual behaviour is like studying any other human behaviour. It requires an objective perspective and an open mind. The only rigorous scientific way to get a group that is truly representative of the Australian population is to take a random sample of people from across the country. The results presented in this book are based on just such a sample of Australians.

What a telephone survey cannot tell us, however, is about the hearts and minds of Australians: what they feel about sex, what it means to them and why they do what they do. To explore these deeper questions, we use in-depth research with methods such as open-ended interviewing. Such research is necessarily done with much smaller numbers of people, but it helps to shed light on what survey findings mean. We have used our experience of such in-depth research when we interpret the survey findings.

A number of case studies or vignettes are presented in boxes in the book. These are composite stories made up by the authors, based on the findings of the national sex survey, plus other research reports and published work. They are designed to illustrate how some of the raw facts translate into everyday experiences.

Juliet Richters and
Chris Rissel, 2005

first times

What does 'having sex' mean? People's first memories of sex range from playing mummies and daddies behind the back shed to a heavily meaning- ful kiss with a first boyfriend or girlfriend. For most people, the defining act that makes you no longer a 'virgin' is vaginal inter- course—whether or not it was the best or the sexiest early sexual experience. In this chapter we look at people's first times, both intercourse and oral sex. By

For most people, it is vaginal intercourse that makes you no longer a 'virgin'—whether or not it was the best early sexual experience.

oral sex we mean fellatio (penis in mouth) and cunnilingus (mouth on vaginal area). We've chosen these sexual acts not because we think they are necessarily what counts as 'having sex', but because they are definable acts that people can mostly remember doing for the first time.

How old are people when they have sex for the first time?

Young people today start having sex earlier than their parents did. Of the people now aged in their fifties, only half the men and less than half the women had vaginal intercourse at age eighteen or earlier. Half the women now in their fifties had intercourse before they turned twenty (i.e. at nineteen or younger). Of the generation now in their early twenties, about half had their first intercourse before their 17th birthday (see Figure 1.1).

People who continue longer in full-time education and go to university are likely to start having sex later than people who are unemployed, working or at technical college. Only about half of first-year university students aged eighteen or nineteen have had sex. It's still a minority of young Australians—around

20 per cent—who have sex before they turn sixteen. A further 30 per cent of young Australians 'lose their virginity' before they turn seventeen.

Having vaginal intercourse (as distinct from sex more broadly) for the first time can mean very different things to different people. It's more likely to be a sexually satisfying event for the male, for whom it is also more likely to be a source of pride than shame. A New Zealand study found that girls who had sex younger were more likely to have been coerced and were more likely to regret it. If we compared first orgasmic sexual encounters rather than first intercourse, the males and females might have more similar feelings.

Figure 1.1 Median age at first vaginal intercourse by year of birth (A median age at first intercourse of 18 means that 50 per cent of people had intercourse when aged 18 or younger.)

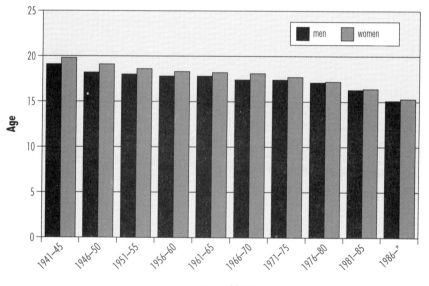

Year of birth

*Note that many of the people in the youngest age group (born since 1986) have not yet had first intercourse, so when they become sexually active the median age for this group will rise.

Source: Rissel et al. 2003, *ANZJPH*, p. 134.

Men who identified as gay when they completed the survey first had intercourse with a woman later than straight men. Some gay men—but only a minority (40 per cent)—had never had sex with a woman at all.

What's the youngest?

There are always a few people who start really early. Some of those who had intercourse for the first time when they were very young (say twelve or younger) were sexually abused, and some had childhood sexual play that included intercourse. The youngest age for first vaginal intercourse reported in this survey was seven.

People who had intercourse for the first time before they turned sixteen were more likely than those who started later to:

- have had sex with more people in their lifetime
- have had oral sex
- have tried anal sex
- have had sex with a same-sex partner
- identify as bisexual
- have had a sexually transmitted infection

What's the oldest?

The oldest age at which anyone in the survey had vaginal intercourse for the first time was fifty-three. Judging from the spread of ages at first intercourse, it seems that someone who has not 'done it' by the time they are thirty is more likely never to do so than to start at a later age.

In the survey, 6 per cent of men and women had never had intercourse (and 2 per cent would not tell us whether they had), but more than half of these people were under twenty and are likely to go on to do it later. About 3 per cent of people never have vaginal intercourse in their lifetimes. A minority of these people are gay men or lesbians who have had no intercourse with an opposite-sex partner.

Which comes first, oral sex or intercourse?

Intercourse comes first for most people. For the older respondents, both men and women, there was typically a gap of six years between first vaginal intercourse and the first time they had oral sex (either fellatio or cunnilingus). Younger men are more likely to have their first experience of intercourse and oral sex in about the same time period. Younger women typically have their first experience of oral sex about a year after first intercourse. About 43 per cent of young men and 31 per cent of young women under twenty have oral sex before they have intercourse for the first time. This is true of only 1 per cent of the respondents in their fifties. For many young people, oral sex does not count as having 'real sex' (see Chapter 5, 'Attitudes towards sex').

In the 1960s, the 'script' or usual pattern for young people experimenting with sex went from first base (kissing), to second base (touching above the waist), to third base (touching below the waist) and only then—if the girl allowed it—to home base or intercourse. Nowadays it seems that for many people the pattern of accepted activities includes oral sex as third base. For other people oral sex is still an additional variation, a more sophisticated extension of the sexual repertoire.

> At 16, Jeremy has finally gone 'all the way'. Half of his friends had already done it (or so they said) and he had been bursting to do it himself. 'Bursting' pretty well described how quickly it happened—he came in about half a minute and it felt like he'd filled up the condom! But it was great, better even than his previous experiences.
>
> He had been out with a few girls before and been with his current girlfriend Kate for about eight months. They had spent a lot of time kissing and touching. The first time she had made him come they'd been at a party and she had stroked his dick with her hand while they sat on a bed in the back room. They'd even been naked together once when his parents had gone out. He'd made her come by rubbing her clit with his hands and then she had sucked him off. It had been fantastic, and since then he'd thought about little else other than what actual intercourse would be like.
>
> He can't wait to tell his friends, although he isn't sure if Kate would like him telling everyone.

Who do people have sex with the first time?

Men are more likely to have intercourse for the first time with a casual partner, whereas women are more likely to have it with their husband, fiancé or steady partner. Only men (mostly older men) reported that their first experience of vaginal intercourse was with a sex worker.

Men tend to have known their first sex partner for a shorter time than women. Older men are more likely than younger men to have had sex for the first time with their wife or fiancée (13 per cent among men in their fifties, but 2 per cent among men in their twenties). Among women in their fifties, 38 per cent had sex for the first time with their husband or fiancé, but only 6 per cent of women in their twenties did so.

Men tend to have known their first sex partner for a shorter time than women.

Men typically have sex for the first time with someone around the same age as themselves, but women are more likely to have sex the first time with someone older than themselves.

Using contraception

There has been a large and steady increase in the use of contraception during first intercourse, from less than 30 per cent of people in the 1950s to over 90 per cent in the 2000s.

In the 1960s and 70s, much of the increase in contraceptive use involved female methods, including the pill. Indeed, the use of condoms at first intercourse went down slightly during the 1960s. From the early 1980s condom use increased rapidly, probably as a result of AIDS awareness and sexual health education in schools. About three-quarters of people now use a condom the first time they have sex. Teenagers starting out are likely to be somewhat younger than their parents were when they had sex for the first time, but today's teenagers are far more likely to do it safely.

Table 1.1 First vaginal intercourse: age of partner

Age of partner	Men (%)	Women (%)
5+ years older	7	14
1–5 years older	23	62
Same age	43	21
1–5 years younger	27	4
5+ years younger	1	0

Source: Rissel et al. 2003, ANZJPH, p. 134.

Teenagers starting out are likely to be somewhat younger than their parents were when they had sex for the first time, but today's teenagers are far more likely to do it safely.

First homosexual experience

Men and women who have a same-sex experience that includes genital contact (6 per cent of women and 5 per cent of men) tend to have this experience later than when most people have vaginal sex for the first time. Men are likely to have a homosexual experience earlier than women—half of the men who had a homosexual experience had it by the time they were nineteen, compared to age twenty-one for women.

Nearly half the women who have had a same-sex experience had their first sexual experience with another woman after the age of twenty-one. This suggests these experiences are part of a more adventurous adult sex life rather than youthful experimentation. This is confirmed by the fact that most of these women continue to see themselves as heterosexual (see Chapter 8, 'Gay and straight'). However, some women may turn to other women after unsatisfactory experiences with men.

Figure 1.2 Use of contraception at first intercourse reported by men and women

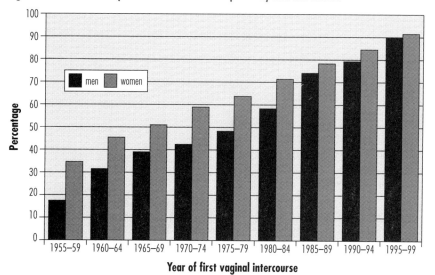

Year of first vaginal intercourse

Source: Rissel et al. 2003, *ANZJPH*, p. 135.

Teenagers

Although young people start their sexual careers a little earlier than people did fifty years ago, the media representation of teenagers as uninhibited and sexually hyperactive is misleading. Older people seem to like to reflect nostalgically on their own sexual desire as adolescents frustrated by the restrictions of earlier times, and they imagine the teenagers of today as having a sexual free-for-all. This fantasy about sex among the young can easily turn to moral panic about the deleterious effects of sex education, the risks of teenage pregnancy or the dangers of sexual abuse. The reality, however, is that compared with people in their twenties and thirties, adolescents have less sex, more anxiety and more embarrassment.

First sexual experiences are rarely the best part of one's sexual life, and most people need practice before sex gets good. Sex, like cooking and driving, needs to be learnt. Books can help but real-life experience is essential.

what people do

What someone is likely to do sexually varies from partner to partner, and from early to late in a relationship. Sex on holiday in a hotel room may be much more elaborate than an early-morning quickie before work on Wednesday. Therefore, what the survey can show us about the variety of sexual activities that Australians engage in is at best a snapshot. This chapter summarises the sexual practices people have ever done and what they did the last time they had sex in the year before their interview.

We've divided the chapter into encounters between men and women and same-sex encounters. This does not necessarily tell you anything about the sexual identity of the participants (see Chapter 8, 'Gay and straight') as a gay man and a lesbian can have a sexual encounter with each other, just as a heterosexual person can have a same-sex encounter.

Encounters between men and women

As mentioned in Chapter 1, the key act that defines 'having sex' for many people is vaginal intercourse. All but 5 per cent of the people who have ever had any sexual contact with a person of the opposite sex have had intercourse. It is what people do most often: 95 per cent of people had intercourse as part of their most recent heterosexual encounter.

Manual sex

Most people said that during their last sexual encounter the man stimulated the woman with his hand (see Table 2.1). The majority

Table 2.1 Sexual practices at most recent encounter with an opposite-sex partner

	Men %	Women %
Vaginal intercourse	96	94
Manual stimulation of woman by man	81	76
Manual stimulation of man by woman	74	70
Cunnilingus	30	24
Fellatio	26	24
Anal intercourse	1	1
Orgasm	95	69

Source: De Visser et al. 2003, *ANZJPH*, p. 152.

> **It is possible that when the last sexual contact consisted only of a grope or a fondle which did not lead to intercourse, people did not regard this as 'having sex'.**

also said that the woman stimulated the man's penis with her hand. We refer to this as 'manual sex', because the formal term 'mutual masturbation' is confusing (does it mean simultaneously?) and we like to keep the word 'masturbation' for what people do to themselves (see Chapter 6, 'Fun for one') rather than what they do to each other.

In both cases, men are more likely than women to say they had manual sex, whether they do it to their female partner or she does it to them. Perhaps the discrepancy is because women are more likely to think that there was so little manual sex (which many people think of as 'foreplay', rather than sex itself) that it didn't count. Or perhaps women are just more shy about saying they have done this. Of course, it is possible that when the last sexual contact consisted only of a grope or a fondle which did not lead to intercourse, people did not regard this as 'having sex'.

Oral sex

Although the majority of people (79 per cent of men and 67 per cent of women) have had oral sex at least once, this is not something most people do every time they have sex. About one person in four had cunnilingus—i.e. oral sex with the man's mouth on the woman's vaginal area—at their last sexual encounter. A similar proportion had fellatio—the woman had gone down on the man—the last time they had sex.

Men are more likely to say they went down on a woman than women are to report that the man went down on them. You might think that if both men and women are telling the truth, the numbers should match exactly. Part of the difference, however, is due to more men having younger partners. An eighteen-year-old man with a fifteen-year-old girlfriend (who is too young to be in the survey) is more likely to have oral sex than a 58-year-old woman with a 62-year-old husband who is too old to be in the survey.

There's a much bigger difference between men and women in the percentages who say they've *ever* had oral sex. This implies that men whose regular partners are not into oral sex are more likely to have had an occasional experience of it with someone else. Or maybe men report a brief experiment as having done it, whereas women don't count this unless it is a

doing it down under

regular part of their sexual repertoire. It's also possible women are minimising, and men exaggerating, their sexual experience when speaking to the interviewer (see discussion of this phenomenon in Appendix 1: The survey).

It seems there has been a change in attitudes towards oral sex over the years. Among people under twenty, exactly the same proportion of men and women say they have had oral sex at some time. Although people in their fifties are just as likely as younger people to have had intercourse, they are less likely—especially the women—to have had oral sex. This is

The early advice books acknowledged that it was more difficult for women to achieve orgasm through intercourse than for men.

probably a remnant of a view from earlier generations that oral sex was deviant, if not depraved—the sort of thing a sex worker would do, but not appropriate for respectable people.

This view is reflected in the older marriage manuals, some of which refer to coitus (vaginal intercourse) as 'the' sex act, and allude to oral sex only obliquely and in passing as 'the genital kiss'. Given the concern still apparent in the mid-twentieth century that it was perverted to reach orgasm by any means other than intercourse, even manual sex to orgasm was under a cloud, let alone oral sex. The early advice books acknowledged that it was more difficult for women to achieve orgasm through intercourse than for men, yet the authors were reluctant to explicitly recommend other sexual practices as a solution to the 'problem'. This was seen as a deficiency of women's anatomy or function rather than as a question of what was okay to do in bed. Alex Comfort's influential book *The Joy of Sex*, first published in 1972, takes a quite different line: 'most people now know that they [genital kisses] are one of the best things in sexual intimacy' (page 137). It is often suggested that higher standards of personal hygiene since the early twentieth century have made oral sex more appealing.

Anal sex

Twenty-five years ago, it might have been difficult for us to ask about anal sex in the survey. Anal intercourse has only become mentionable since the AIDS epidemic burst onto the pages of our newspapers in the early 1980s. Before then, at least in English-speaking countries, it was something that was occasionally darkly referred to as a 'vice' or hinted at in the reports of divorce cases where the wife complained that the husband subjected her to 'deviant practices'. However, anal sex has always been around and many recent surveys have shown that it is practised among both homosexuals and heterosexuals all around the world.

Only a minority of people—21 per cent of men and 15 per cent of women—have ever had anal intercourse with an opposite-sex partner. Even for people who have tried anal sex, it is not something they do regularly: less than 1 per cent did it the last time they had sex.

Combinations of practices

The most common sexual encounter between men and women consists of the partners stimulating each other's genitals by hand, followed (or preceded) by vaginal intercourse. Figure 2.1 shows that at their most recent sexual encounter, about half the respondents had intercourse plus manual stimulation of either or both partners, about a third had intercourse plus manual plus oral sex (given and/or received), and 12 per cent had only intercourse. Only around 7 per cent had any other combination, including 'none of the above' (i.e. they had sex but not any of the practices we asked about), oral or manual sex without vaginal intercourse and any combination including anal sex.

Figure 2.1 Combinations of sexual practices at most recent encounter with an opposite-sex partner

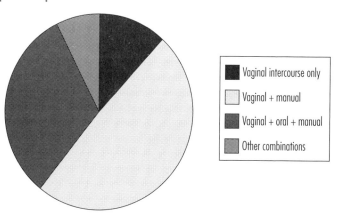

Vaginal intercourse only

Vaginal + manual

Vaginal + oral + manual

Other combinations

Other practices

Of course there are many more things that people may have done together at their last sexual encounter that we did not ask about: hugging, kissing, 'dry rooting', stroking, stimulating their own genitals, sucking breasts, playing with fruit or sex toys, spanking—the list is endless. Later in the questionnaire, we asked whether people had done some of these things in the last year, and the results are shown in Chapter 7, 'Kinky stuff'. Some people (less than 1 per cent) had done none of the things we asked about last time they had sex.

Orgasm

It is unusual for a man not to have an orgasm when he has sex with a woman: only 5 per cent of men in the survey did not reach orgasm the last time they had sex. But it's much more common for women: 31 per cent did not come at their last sexual encounter. This difference is reflected in Chapter 13, 'Sexual difficulties', where we note that women were much more likely than men to have trouble reaching orgasm.

One reason for this is perhaps the heavy concentration on intercourse as the central, almost compulsory sexual practice, which is more effective as a way for men to reach orgasm than for women. This guess is confirmed when we look at the relationship between what people did at their last sexual encounter and whether they came (see Tables 2.2 and 2.3). Here we ignore whether people gave oral or manual stimulation to the partner, and look only at what the partner did to them, i.e. cunnilingus for women and fellatio for men.

In general men were highly likely to have an orgasm in any encounter that included vaginal intercourse, but were somewhat less likely to come if they only had oral and/or manual sex.

Women who have frequent orgasms are more likely to be satisfied with their sex lives.

Nonetheless, among men whose partners stimulated them manually or went down on them as well, more than 80 per cent had an orgasm. In contrast, women who had vaginal intercourse but nothing else had only a 50 per cent chance of reaching orgasm. Among those who had intercourse and whose partners also stimulated them manually—the largest group—71 per cent had an orgasm. If their partners went down on them as well, 86 per cent had an orgasm. Among women who only received manual sex, 79 per cent had an orgasm. Few people had anal intercourse, but it did not seem to make much difference to the likelihood of orgasm for men or women.

We cannot assume, of course, that everyone having sex wants to reach orgasm every time. Although women who have frequent orgasms are more likely to be satisfied with their sex lives, it does not matter to everyone whether they have an orgasm on every occasion of sex. Women in the survey who had sex more often in the past four weeks were also more likely to have an orgasm the last time they had sex.

Table 2.2 Combinations of sexual practices and orgasm at men's most recent encounter with a female partner

Sexual practices	Proportion of men who did this (%)	Proportion of men who reached orgasm (%)
Vaginal intercourse only	23	95
Intercourse + manual*	48	95
Intercourse + oral**	2	99
Intercourse + oral + manual	22	98
Manual only	2	82
Manual + oral	2	87
Oral only	0	–
Any combination, including anal	1	98

* Manual stimulation by female partner
** Oral stimulation by female partner (fellatio)

Table 2.3 Combinations of sexual practices and orgasm at women's most recent encounter with a male partner

Sexual practices	Proportion of women who did this (%)	Proportion of women who reached orgasm (%)
Vaginal only	20	50
Vaginal + manual*	53	71
Vaginal + oral**	3	73
Vaginal + oral + manual	21	86
Manual only	2	79
Manual + oral	1	90
Oral only	<1	79
Any combination including anal	1	71

* Manual stimulation by male partner
** Oral stimulation by male partner (cunnilingus)

Jackie and Peter were what most people considered a cosy couple. They'd been living together for a few years and both could see themselves settling down together. The sex was mostly satisfying, although Jackie didn't always feel like doing it. The last time they'd done it had been quite good, and Peter had been quite attentive, even going down on her. She liked that even though he could do with some more practice! He was always good with his hands and liked to stroke and massage her, and could reliably bring her to orgasm with his hands and fingers. They had a few favourite positions—her on top, the 'missionary position'—and he liked to come when they were in the 'doggy' position (him inside her from behind). If they had time they'd try a few other positions. She'd never tried anal sex and wasn't that interested, but sometimes wondered what a vibrator would be like.

Same-sex encounters

More women (9 per cent) than men (6 per cent) report some form of same-sex experience in their lifetime. However, if only genital contact is counted, the proportion of men (5 per cent) and women (6 per cent) having a same-sex experience is similar. Here we do not distinguish between whether people think of themselves as homosexual (gay or lesbian) or not, simply note that they have had some same-sex interaction.

Table 2.4 Sexual practices at most recent encounter with a same-sex partner

	Men (%)	Women (%)
Manual stimulation of respondent	89	95
Manual stimulation of partner	90	91
Oral sex – receiving	75	66
Oral sex – giving	76	62
Anal intercourse – insertive	38	n.a.*
Anal intercourse – receptive	30	n.a.*
Orgasm	89	76

* n.a. means not applicable

Anal stimulation or insertion by fingers or dildos not asked

Source: Grulich et al. 2003, ANZJPH, p. 161.

On the last occasion of sex with someone of the same sex, most people said they stimulated their partner with their hands and were stimulated in return (see Table 2.4). Three out of four of these encounters by men involved fellatio, both giving and receiving, and two out of three women having sex with another woman engaged in cunnilingus.

Oral sex is much more common in homosexual interactions than in heterosexual interactions. Women having sex with other women are also more likely to reach orgasm than when they have sex with men. The opposite is true for men in a homosexual encounter, with fewer men reaching orgasm than in a heterosexual encounter. This seems to indicate that if you want to be sure of reaching orgasm next time you have sex, you have a better chance if you have sex with a woman—whichever sex you are.

It is plausible that women are better at stimulating other women and doing 'what works'. But it seems surprising that men should not also be better at doing what other men enjoy best. However, one reason for the lower orgasm rate in male–male encounters might be that the encounters would include more casual and anonymous sex. Thus men may have more brief or partial encounters with no opportunity for both men to reach orgasm. From other studies we know that men have more opportunities to have casual and anonymous sex than women do. In sex clubs, gay saunas and even in some parks and toilets men can find other men willing to have sex without strings attached, often without any conversation.

> **If you want to be sure of reaching orgasm next time you have sex, you have a better chance if you have sex with a woman—whichever sex you are.**

Anal sex

Not surprisingly, anal sex is more common among men in a homosexual interaction than in heterosexual encounters. About 40 per cent of men had anal intercourse in their most recent homosexual interaction, compared to 1 per cent for the most recent heterosexual encounter. But anal intercourse is by no means a universal practice in sex between men. Men having sex with each other are more likely to use their hands and mouths than to have anal intercourse.

3 how often

It is commonly said that men think about sex every eight seconds, or something equally silly. This seems to be a statistic invented by a bored journalist in a bar. If it were true, how would men have time to think about anything else, such as football? And how do people know exactly how often they think about sex? What counts as thinking about sex—a full-scale fantasy of having sex with someone, or just a fleeting thought about something vaguely related to sex? For these reasons we didn't even try to ask the question in our survey. However, the United States national sex survey in 1992 did ask 'How often do you think about sex?' They found that men said they thought about sex more often than women did—more than half the men said they thought about sex 'every day' or 'several times a day', whereas the majority of women said they thought about it 'a few times a week' or 'a few times a month'. We're inclined to suspect that men and women count different things as 'thinking about sex'. We'd have to talk to lots of people to find out for sure, but it's likely that every time a man sees a woman cross the road and thinks 'Oh, she's attractive', he would count that as 'thinking about sex'. A woman looking at an attractive man probably wouldn't.

> **It's likely that every time a man sees a woman cross the road and thinks 'Oh, she's attractive', he would count that as 'thinking about sex'.**

How often do people want to have sex?

We asked everyone, even those who were not currently having sex, how often they would ideally like to have sex. The answers ranged from never to more than once a day. Although men, on average, want sex more often than women, the difference between them is not very large. Most people, men or women, want sex a few times a week. The main difference between men and women is that nearly a quarter of the men want sex at least daily, and only 8 per cent of the women want sex daily or more often. Perhaps women are more concerned with quality than quantity?

Figure 3.1 Preferred frequency of sex

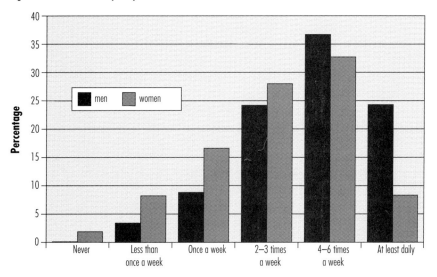

Source: Richters et al. 2003, *ANZJPH*, p. 176.

Although only a tiny proportion of people—less than 1 per cent—said they 'never' wanted to have sex, about 3 per cent refused to answer the question or said they didn't know. It's probably very difficult for people, especially men, to say that they don't want sex at all.

How often do people really have sex?

We asked people how often they'd actually had sex with any partner in the past four weeks, and then converted the answers into times per week. (We have not tried to compare same-sex couples with heterosexual couples. Less than half a per cent of men and less than 1 per cent of women in the survey are in regular homosexual relationships, and any statistics based on such a small group of people would not be very reliable.) Unfortunately, reality does not correspond with what people ideally want.

The majority of people have sex less than twice a week. That means most people are getting less sex than they want—or would ideally prefer. Of course, we don't know whether all the extra sex they ideally want would be with

Most people are getting less sex than they want—or would ideally prefer. Although on average men say they have sex more often than women, the difference is not large.

their current partner or with someone else. Although on average men say they have sex more often than women, the difference is not large compared to how often people would ideally like to have sex.

Figure 3.2 Actual frequency of sex in the past four weeks

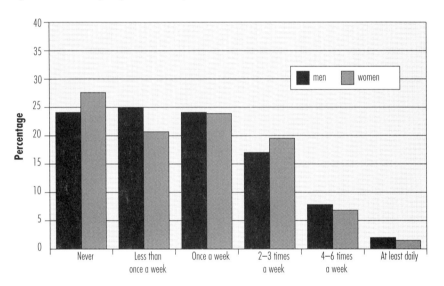

Source: Richters et al. 2003, *ANZJPH*, p. 176.

The majority of people—86 per cent of men and 69 per cent of women—seem to want sex more often than they are having it. How do people cope with this? Not surprisingly, people who want more sex are more likely to masturbate than those who get enough or too much. (See Chapter 6, 'Fun for one', for other things that people do to substitute for sex or to add sexual interest.)

Only 1 per cent of all men say they want sex less often than they have it. But here's a curious fact: there's one age group where 8 per cent of men appear to want less sex than they are getting—men under twenty. Maybe some young men are not as sexually insatiable as everyone makes out, or maybe they exaggerate about how often they really have sex.

Around 6 per cent of women said they wanted less sex than they were getting, but only 3 per cent of the under-twenties said this. Interestingly, women under twenty were less likely than women in their twenties, thirties or forties to say that sex in their relationship was 'extremely' physically pleasurable (see Chapter 9, 'Domestic bliss'). So if the sex isn't all that fantastic, why do they want more of it? (Perhaps they know that practice makes perfect.)

At 29, Sarah enjoys her sex life. She has a good job as a sales manager, is paying off the mortgage on her own flat, and feels she generally knows what she wants. It wasn't always like that. During her late teens, she started going out with boys and had a few close boyfriends. But they were all so keen to get their own rocks off they hadn't much time to please her; sometimes they even hurt her during sex. As she got older and got to know her own body better, and her partners got older and more experienced, she found she really enjoyed sex.

Sex with Ian, her current partner, has been great, especially when they first started seeing each other. They didn't leave her flat for a whole long weekend the first time he stayed over. He was thirty and she was thinking in the back of her mind that he might be the one she would settle down with if he asked her.

After going out with Ian for almost three years, Sarah has worked out that on average they have sex only once or twice a week because his job is so full-on and there are often evening meetings and business trips he is expected to go on. Sarah finds it a bit funny that she wants sex more often than Ian seems to. She is pretty close to her mother so she mentioned it to her. Her mother admitted that she too sometimes wanted more sex than Sarah's father, but had never told anyone before. Her own mother—Sarah's grandmother—had taught her that men 'only wanted one thing' and that you had to let them do it occasionally, but you mustn't make yourself 'cheap'.

The biggest influence on whether you get sex when you want it is whether you have someone to have sex with.

The biggest influence on whether you get sex when you want it is whether you have someone to have sex with. Figure 3.3 shows that people without a regular partner are most likely not to have had sex in the past four weeks or have it less than once a week. If they do have sex, it may be with a casual partner or, for a few people, with a regular partner they broke up with during the past month. Regular partners who do not live together have sex more often than people who live together. One reason is that they are likely to be younger. Another is that if people in a relationship stop having sex, they are likely not to report their friend as a 'regular sexual partner' if they are not living together. But a couple who live together may go on regarding themselves as in a sexual relationship even if they have not had sex for weeks or months.

'Not now, the kids will hear us!'

Is there sex after children? Usually the arrival of a baby reduces the frequency of sex. For some couples the pregnancy is a major turn-on. For others, sex may become less frequent as the pregnancy progresses and then stop altogether for a time, depending upon how the birth went and whether there were any tears or stitches. On top of that exhaustion and coping with the demands of a totally dependent infant can certainly interrupt

Figure 3.3 Frequency of sex in the past four weeks among people with or without regular partners

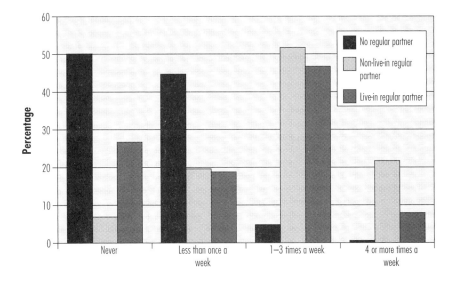

the romance and leisurely lovemaking couples may have had before a baby.

Once a couple gets over the incredible event of childbirth and a child is added to the dynamics of their relationship, what happens to the frequency of sex? In our survey about half of the adults (47 per cent) lived in a household with children under 16 years old. More women (50 per cent) than men (45 per cent) lived with at least one child. What happens to the frequency of sex once the children get older? To answer these questions we need to focus first on people who are in a regular sexual relationship and living together. Then we can compare how often people with and without children have sex. We also need to take into account people's ages, because on average, older people have sex less often.

Table 3.1 shows the basic pattern of how often people living with an opposite-sex partner have sex, depending on whether they have children and the ages of the children. The table does not take into account the age of the adults.

Table 3.1 Frequency of sex with live-in opposite-sex partner in the past four weeks

Family type	Frequency of sex in the past four weeks (%)			
	Never	Less than once a week	1–3 times a week	4 or more times a week
No children	31	16	41	12
One child under five years	25	21	46	8
One child between five and fifteen years	28	21	44	7
Two or more children under five years	25	21	47	6
Two children between five and fifteen years	29	16	46	9
Three or more children between five and fifteen years	23	18	48	11
Children under five and between five and fifteen years	22	20	48	10

The presence of children, whether younger or older or some combination of ages, does not seem to make much difference to how often the adults have sex. If anything, the couples without children were the most likely to have had no sex in the past four weeks. However, the no-children category also includes a sizeable group having sex very often (more than four times a week), and this might be because these people are younger. It also doesn't seem to make a big difference how many children there are. Indeed, people with three or more children seem to be as likely as other couples to have sex four or more times a week. This is perhaps not so surprising in light of the fact that children are a by-product of sexual activity.

When we make a statistical adjustment to allow for the age of the couple, there is only one change to our conclusion about the effect of the presence of children on the average frequency of sex. This change is that people with one child under five years of age have sex less often than other people. This will come as no surprise for new parents with their first child! The good news is that your sex life should return to normal, at least as far as frequency is concerned.

The couples without children were the most likely to have had no sex in the past four weeks.

Our survey was cross-sectional, a one-off 'slice of time'. The best way to follow the effects of having children on people's sex lives is to survey the same people repeatedly over several years. There is another study currently in progress that will tell us more about changes in people's sex lives over time.

how many partners

At some point in a relationship, usually early or after the 'first time', the conversation will turn to: 'So, how many people have you slept with before me?' Your partner's experience can raise sensitive issues about how you compare ('Am I as good or good enough?') and questions about what your partner might expect of you during sex. There is also a health concern. Generally speaking, people with more sexual partners are more likely to have had a sexually transmitted infection in their life, especially if they have had unsafe sex. These days the question of an HIV test also comes up (see Chapter 16, 'Sexually transmitted infections and safe sex').

The popular impression from television serials, movies and magazines is that everyone is having sex with lots of people. In real life serial monogamy is most common, with someone breaking up with their regular partner and then pairing up with someone else. This reality is very different from what is displayed in the popular media, where concurrent partners or 'affairs' are often the basis of television or movie dramas (see Chapter 10, 'Is your partner cheating on you?').

> **The popular impression from television serials, movies and magazines is that everyone is having sex with lots of people.**

According to the survey, heterosexual men have had sex, on average, with about seventeen female partners (regular or casual) in their lives so far. Heterosexual women have had sex with about seven males. Somewhat surprisingly, bisexual and lesbian women had, on average, about three times as many male sexual partners as heterosexual women. Perhaps this is because heterosexual women are more likely to settle down with a man, but women with lesbian inclinations may try several men before they are convinced that straight sex is not for them. Also, gay and bisexual people generally have more liberal sexual values than straight people, so lesbians and bi-sexual women who mix in queer circles in the inner city may find their friends much less likely to disapprove of casual sex than their married relatives in the suburbs. Gay men mostly have far fewer female sexual partners than straight men, but bisexual men have the same or more.

Lesbians are more similar to straight women than to gay men when it comes to the number of sexual partners they have. The lesbians we surveyed had on average about eight female partners in their lives so far, and one in the past year.

On the other hand the average number of male partners for gay men is a whopping 79 over their lifetime and eleven in the past year. However, these averages are affected by the very high numbers of partners that some gay men have—some have thousands of same-sex partners, but this is quite rare. In the past year, 21 per cent of gay men had no partners at all, and a further 35 per cent only had one or two. Gay and bisexual men were less likely to be in a regular relationship than other people, and this meant that they could clock up large numbers of one-off partners without necessarily having sex any more often than other people.

Charlie, 38, came home from drinks with his long-time mate Dave. They'd met at TAFE when they were training to be electricians and knew each other pretty well. They'd been through each others' various relationships, engagements, marriages and kids. Dave was now sepa-rated and about to be back on the singles scene—hence the night out. Charlie knew of about ten women Dave had been with since they'd been friends, including his now ex-wife, and he figured there'd been a few before they met. Charlie assumed Dave had had sex with those ten women and was mildly envious that Dave would be out there again, notching up a few more.

Charlie himself had been an early starter. If he counted half a dozen encounters with women that were very passionate and quite intimate, but didn't quite end up in the sack the way he'd wanted to, it came to nineteen partners, including Liz, his wife of seventeen years.

Charlie knew Liz had had a few sexual partners before she met him. They'd talked about it early on in their relationship. She'd been a little coy with him, though, and he's never been sure that she'd told him about every single one. Sure, she'd told him about the serious relation-ships and about the guy she'd done it with the first time, but he felt there were still a few mysteries in her past. In the end he shrugged it off—he didn't really want to think about those other guys. He was just glad she was with him.

Opposite-sex partners

A few men and women report hundreds, even thousands, of opposite-sex partners over their lifetime. While this is very rare it does happen. Some people with very high numbers of partners have visited sex workers, or have worked in the sex industry themselves. Others just take every opportunity they can get—they look for people to have sex with at work, on holidays, through the Internet—seeking out situations where casual or anonymous sex is easy to arrange.

A few men and women report hundreds, even thousands, of opposite-sex partners over their lifetime.

Figure 4.1 Lifetime number of opposite-sex partners

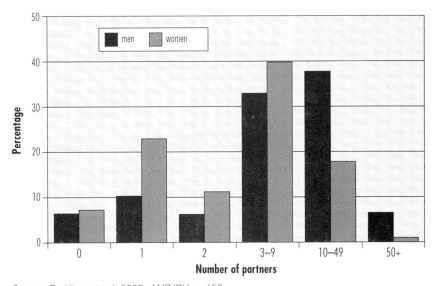

Source: De Visser et al. 2003, *ANZJPH*, p. 150.

More men than women have had very large numbers of partners. The availability of paid sex is one explanation why men on average say they have had more sexual partners than women. Men also have more opportunities to have sex with women who are not strictly speaking sex workers—for example bar girls in some Asian countries may be prepared to have sex in return for dinner and drinks. In some places local men meet women tourists for the same reason, but it is less common. Another major reason for this difference between men and women is that men exaggerate—and women underestimate— the number of partners they've had (see discussion of this in Appendix 1: The survey). Men seem to be more generous about including people in the list—they are more likely to count any sexual contact with a woman as 'sex', while women may only include men they've had intercourse with.

Women seem to present themselves as less sexually active than they really are, perhaps for fear of being labelled 'sluts'. An American study of university students found that women reported smaller numbers of partners when they thought someone would see their questionnaire responses, and larger numbers when they thought they were attached to a lie detector.

In the five years before this interview, straight men had on average four partners and women had two. In the past 12 months straight men had on average one or two female sexual partners and women had one male sexual partner. As you would expect, averages do not fit everyone. Younger people have had fewer partners in their lives than older people, because they have not had time to meet them yet. Young men had more partners in the past year (on average 1.3 partners for men under twenty, and 1.5 for men in their twenties or thirties) than older men, who had on average one partner. Women typi- cally had just one partner in the past year, whatever age they were. In the past year, about three-quarters of men and women had sex with just one person; 15 per cent of men and 9 per cent of women had two or more sexual partners.

The people who are most likely to have two or more sexual partners are young people, single, widowed or divorced people, and people on lower incomes. Women who speak a language other than English at home, people living in remote areas, and managers and professional people were less likely to have had two or more partners in the past year.

People in their forties and fifties are more likely than younger people to have settled down with the first or second person they had sex with. The typical pattern nowadays is for most heterosexuals to have sex with up to ten or so people before settling down in their late twenties or thirties with a long- term partner. Most of these ten or so partners are medium- or long-term relationships, and some are one-off or casual partners. Among the over-forties only a few people each year have sex with more than one person, either because their relationship has broken up and they are 'on the market' again, or because they have sex on the side (see Chapter 10, 'Is your partner cheating on you?').

Same-sex partners

The majority of people who have ever had sex with a same-sex partner are in fact heterosexuals—that is to say, they identify as straight and they mostly have sex with opposite-sex partners. In Figure 4.2, for example, men who identify as gay would be a large proportion of those with high numbers of partners, but a small proportion of those with only one male partner in their lives. Although more women than men have ever had a same-sex partner, it is men who are likely to have high numbers of partners. Many of the men's partners are a result of casual encounters rather than regular relationships. This is reflected in the differences between Figure 4.2 and Figure 4.3.

Figure 4.2 Lifetime number of male partners among men (The 95 per cent of men with no male partners have been omitted from the graph.)

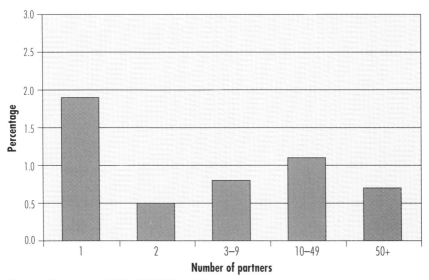

Source: Grulich et al. 2003, *ANZJPH*, p. 158.

Figure 4.3 Lifetime number of female partners among women (The 94 per cent of women with no female partners have been omitted from the graph.)

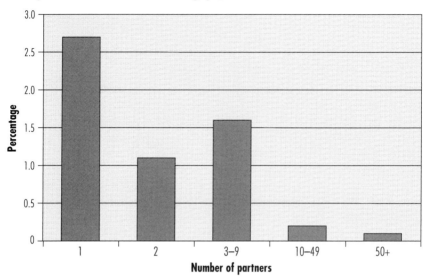

Source: Grulich et al. 2003, *ANZJPH*, p. 159.

attitudes towards sex

How sexually open-minded are Australians? What do they think about casual sex, or homosexual sex? Are women more liberal than men? What about when it comes to pornography? Our findings confirmed the view that people's attitudes towards sex can be complex and not always consistent. Attitudes towards sex may influence behaviour, but behaviour can also influence attitudes. A previously fixed attitude—disapproving of abortion, for example—can be changed by a new experience, such as an unwanted pregnancy. People whose religious views or simple prejudice led them to condemn homosexuality may find themselves rethinking their views if they discover that one of their children is gay.

Society's attitudes towards sex have a historical background that includes the influences of economics, law and colonisation as well as local culture and religion. In poor countries, despite generally restrictive sexual mores, rural families close to starvation may welcome income from daughters doing sex work in the city. A newly settled area with a large male population and few women may be tolerant of sex workers—until families move in. The law is an expression of community values but also in its turn influences what people consider acceptable. For example, teenagers may use the 'age of consent' of 16 (or 17 in South Australia or Tasmania) as a guide to when they 'ought' to have sex for the first time.

Historical change can be rapid, and attitudes change at the same time. In just the past twenty years, the average age at first marriage has risen from 25 to 29 for men and from 22 to 27 for women. The current minimum legal age for marriage in Australia is eighteen, although it is possible to marry at sixteen or seventeen with permission from the parents and from a judge or magistrate. Before amendments to the Marriage Act in 1991, a girl could marry at fourteen with the court's permission. This had become rare long before the Act was changed, but in the days before legal abortion and support payments for single parents, permission might be given if a girl was pregnant and the husband or his family were able to support her financially.

When many of the older people in our survey first became sexually active, abortion was effectively illegal in most states, and therefore expensive and difficult to obtain. Many high school students heard tales of a schoolmate who left school suddenly and went to another city where she lived in a hostel for unmarried mothers until giving birth. Often she surrendered the child for adoption, now a rare option for women experiencing unplanned pregnancy (see Chapter 11, 'Getting pregnant').

How sexually liberal are you?

Try yourself on this quick attitude quiz. If you strongly agree with a statement, put a ring around the number next to 'Strongly agree', and so on. Then add up your score.

1. Films these days are too sexually explicit.

   Strongly agree 1   Agree 2   Neither 3   Disagree 4   Strongly 5
                                  agree nor   disagree
                                  disagree

2. Sex before marriage is acceptable.

   Strongly agree 5   Agree 4   Neither 3   Disagree 2   Strongly 1
                                  agree nor   disagree
                                  disagree

3. Abortion is always wrong.

   Strongly agree 1   Agree 2   Neither 3   Disagree 4   Strongly 5
                                  agree nor   disagree
                                  disagree

4. Having an affair when in a committed relationship is always wrong.

   Strongly agree 1   Agree 2   Neither 3   Disagree 4   Strongly 5
                                  agree nor   disagree
                                  disagree

5. Sex between two adult women is always wrong.

   Strongly agree 1   Agree 2   Neither 3   Disagree 4   Strongly 5
                                  agree nor   disagree
                                  disagree

6. Sex between two adult men is always wrong.

   Strongly agree 1   Agree 2   Neither 3   Disagree 4   Strongly 5
                                  agree nor   disagree
                                  disagree

Total: If you scored

25 or above you are very liberal and broad-minded about sexual issues. You are probably prepared to try new things sexually and have considerable sexual experience. If you're straight you are likely to have some gay friends and you may have experimented with a same-sex partner. You are probably not religious and you probably drink more alcohol than the average person.

between 20 and 24 you are fairly tolerant, though not completely committed to sexual freedom and exploration. Perhaps there is just one thing that you heavily disapprove of, such as sexual infidelity or abortion, while you are strongly in favour of other aspects of a sexually liberal life.

13 to 19 you are middle of the road, sexually speaking. You are not a prude, but you are not the most adventurous person either. Your tolerance of other people's behaviour has limits. People from non-English-speaking backgrounds are more likely to be in this category or the next one than are people who speak English at home.

12 or less you are definitely conservative in your attitudes towards sex. You disapprove of 'recreational sex', especially outside committed heterosexual relationships. You are probably not a risk-taker generally. You are likely to be over 50, to have a religion, to identify as heterosexual and perhaps to avoid sex altogether. If you're a woman, you're more likely to live in the country than in a city.

What do most Australians think about these questions?

Over a third of the survey respondents agreed with the statement 'Films these days are too sexually explicit', with women more likely than men to agree (see Figure 5.1). Sexual imagery on television generally has a generational impact, with younger men and women less likely than older people to believe films are too sexually explicit.

Premarital sex is widely, but not universally, accepted—85 per cent agree it is acceptable, but 11 per cent disagree. Women overall are slightly less likely to accept premarital sex than men. Young men under 20 are less likely than other men to approve of it. Perhaps this is the age group who are most likely to be idealistic about following religious dictates, or perhaps some young people who are nervous about embarking on a sexual relationship think of sex as happening in some distant, safe, married future.

Figure 5.1 Agreement with sexual attitude statements

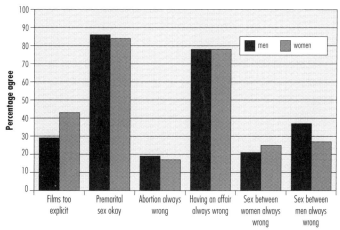

Source: Rissel et al. 2003, *ANZJPH*, p. 119.

Less than one respondent in five agrees with the statement 'Abortion is always wrong'. Women are slightly more liberal than men on this issue. People under twenty are more judgmental, being more likely to agree that abortion is always wrong, but again the differences are small.

The majority of people agree that 'Having an affair when in a committed relationship is always wrong'. This is the only statement where the majority view is counter to a sexually liberal position, even though the statement is uncompromising ('is *always* wrong'). Some people when answering this question may exclude an occasional transgression from their definition of 'affair', or perhaps their understanding of a 'committed relationship' means sex with other people is wrong by definition. It appears that Australians—both men and women equally—are strongly committed to sexual exclusivity in relationships, though as they get older they are less likely to agree it is always wrong to have an affair (see Chapter 10, 'Is your partner cheating on you?').

The responses to the two statements on sex between women and sex between men show that people do not simply condone or condemn homosexual activity. The majority of people do not think same-sex activity is always wrong. In general women are more tolerant than men. Women are also more consistent in their views—about a quarter of women agree homosexual activity is wrong whether it is between men or between

The picture of two women making out together is an appealing fantasy for many men.

women. Men's views, however, are more likely to differ depending on who is having the sex. Men are *more* tolerant than women about sex between women, but they are less tolerant than women about sex between men. Women are more often unsure than men, saying they neither agree nor disagree.

There are various plausible interpretations of the differences between men's and women's views. Heterosexual men may be more disapproving of male same-sex activity because in general men are more sexually aggressive than women, so men—especially teenagers—may fear being the unwilling object of other men's sexual attentions. In contrast, the picture of two women making out together is an appealing fantasy for many men, and it is a popular image in pornography aimed at a male heterosexual audience. Men seem to see this scene as 'two nice girls who would love to have me join them' rather than as a lesbian scene where a man might be unnecessary or unwelcome. For this and other reasons, occasional same-sex activity between women who are otherwise heterosexual is more permissible in Australian society than sex between men. This is borne out in the results in Chapter 8, 'Gay and straight'. More women than men have had some same-sex experience, and women are more likely to regard themselves as heterosexual (rather than bisexual or lesbian) despite having done so. In contrast, many men's ideas of appropriate heterosexual masculinity are so rigid they consider any man who has tried sex with another man just once to be a 'poofter'.

Indeed many people think of any man who has sex with another man as gay, and of any woman who has sex with another woman as lesbian, so for them the questions we asked are equivalent to 'Do you disapprove of gay men and lesbians?' Interpreted in that light, the responses suggest that women are somewhat less likely to be prejudiced against gay men than men are, and that both men and women over fifty are less tolerant of gays and lesbians than younger people.

Is there a generation gap in sexual attitudes?

Despite what we've just said about views on homosexuality, these results do not show a generation gap in Australians' sexual attitudes: in fact the consistency of opinions across age groups was striking. People over fifty are slightly less liberal than other age groups, but the difference is very small, much smaller than the difference between 'Anglo' Australians and those from non-English-speaking backgrounds, or between heterosexuals and non-heterosexuals (bisexuals, gay men and lesbians).

However, the survey only covered people up to 59. The generation gap before and after what has been optimistically called the sexual revolution is probably between the baby boomers—people now in their forties and fifties—and their parents, now in their sixties, seventies and eighties. Try asking your parents or grandparents the questions in the quiz and see how they score!

Maria, 58, is retired and about to become a grandmother. This is wonderful news. She has been looking forward to having a grandchild to spoil. However, she knows that she and her daughter, Helen, who is 31 and works as a legal secretary in a large firm in the city, will be sure to disagree on a number of issues. They just seem to have different views on many things, and Maria understands she is probably what some people would call 'old-fashioned'. She thinks of herself as having decent family values. For example, she does not see the point of having semi-naked women in prime-time movies. She feels uncomfortable about the idea of homosexuality. And she could not believe it when President Clinton tried to argue that he hadn't had sex with 'that woman' when they had obviously been intimate together—he had 'stained' her dress! That was the end of any respect she had for that president.

Maria is glad that Helen is married and believes in being faithful. She isn't sure having too liberal a view is always the best—there has to be some risk involved in being open to every new idea that comes along. She wants her grandchildren to have some basic values that will stand them in good stead for the future.

How important is sex to you?

Together with the attitude statements we asked people for their views on three other statements related to sex. The first was: 'An active sex life is important for your sense of well-being.' Most people—88 per cent of men and 80 per cent of women—agreed with this, with the highest agreement in all age groups over thirty and the lowest in the under twenties. It's likely that until someone has experienced a long-term sexual relationship, they don't have the opportunity to find out how they feel when they do or don't get regular sex.

Sex tends to get better the longer you know someone

Agreeing with this statement indicates a preference for sex in long-term, usually committed, relationships rather than casual sex with a variety of partners. About two thirds of men and women agree with this statement. This is consistent with Australians' values in favour of one-to-one relationships (see Chapter 10, 'Is your partner cheating on you?'). Young people under twenty are often undecided on this question, again perhaps indicating a lack of experience. Women in their fifties are less likely to agree with this statement than women aged 20 to 49. This suggests it is possible to know someone for too long—the benefit of longer acquaintance does not increase indefinitely.

The Clinton question

If two people had oral sex, but not intercourse, would you still consider that they had had sex together? Overall, 72 per cent of Australians count oral sex as 'sex', but many young people take former President Bill Clinton's view and disagree. Only 46 per cent of young men under twenty and 37 per cent of young women count oral sex as sex, and a further 10 per cent of young women are unsure. Surveys of Australian university students have found similar results. It is possible that HIV prevention campaigns that emphasised the use of condoms since the mid-1980s may have fostered the view that the only 'real' sex is the sort you use a condom for. At the same time, oral sex has become a more accepted part of people's sexual repertoire: younger people are more likely to have oral sex (nearly half of women over fifty have never had oral sex at all), and about a third of the youngest age group in the survey had oral sex before they had vaginal intercourse for the first time (see Chapter 1, 'First times').

A third of the youngest age group in the survey had oral sex before they had vaginal intercourse for the first time.

6 fun for one

Wanking, touching or playing with yourself, jerking off, spanking the monkey, beating your meat, tossing off, self-service, 'working on finding my G spot', feeding the chooks—there are dozens of terms for it, both Australian and imported—though many seem to refer specifically to male masturbation. Does everyone masturbate? Well, no.

Only two thirds of the men and one third of the women in the survey masturbated alone in the past year. Half of the men and 20 per cent of the women masturbated in the past four weeks. As well as being more likely to masturbate, men do it more often: half of those who masturbated in the past four weeks did it more than once a week. And 1.5 per cent of men did it daily or more often.

People with more education and people who live in cities are more likely to masturbate than less educated people and people who live in the country. Gay, lesbian and bisexual people are much more likely to masturbate than straight people. These differences suggest that wanting to masturbate is not only a matter of how randy you feel but also a matter of your sexual values and attitudes: more liberal people are more ready to do so, or at least are more ready to admit it in an interview.

Wanting to masturbate is not only a matter of how randy you feel but also a matter of your sexual values and attitudes.

Both men and women in their fifties masturbate less, but it is even more noticeable that women under twenty are the least likely to masturbate. Some sex therapists express concern that young women's reluctance to explore their own bodies—despite reaching puberty earlier than boys—deprives them of know-ledge about their own sexual responses. This may contribute to the lesser physical enjoyment young women tend to have in partnered sex compared with young men (see Chapter 9, 'Domestic bliss').

Figure 6.1 Masturbation in the past year

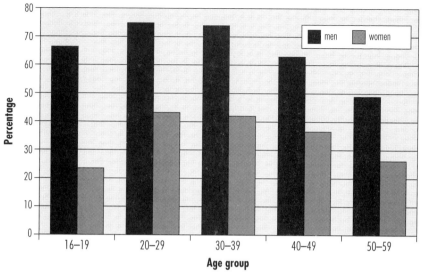

Source: Richters et al. 2003, ANZJPH, p. 184.

Traditionally, some cultures have regarded masturbation as dangerous—either mentally ('it'll make you an idiot, soft in the head') or physically ('you'll go blind', 'it weakens your health', 'your hair will fall out and you'll get cancer'). However, these ideas received no support from scientific medicine or psychology during the twentieth century. Masturbation is now generally regarded by the medical profession, by sex researchers and by sex therapists as common and harmless—even desirable. Certainly it's much safer than having unprotected sex with a stranger, and much cheaper than visiting a sex worker.

There's nothing wrong with *not* masturbating, however. Some people just don't feel like sex without a partner.

Aren't people too embarrassed to answer about masturbation?

It seems not, at least not on the telephone. Only 2 per cent of men and 5 per cent of women refused to answer this question. More people refused to tell us their income. It's also possible that some people just said they didn't masturbate rather than ask the interviewer exactly what counted as 'masturbating'. If anyone doing the survey asked the interviewer whether it still counted as masturbation if you didn't have an orgasm, the interviewer said it did. But it's likely that many people do not count stimulating themselves as masturbating unless they come. Some people may not have wanted to risk being asked by the interviewer to give further details about how or when they did it. It's possible, too, that women are genuinely less clear than men about what counts as masturbation, such as self-stimulation by rubbing against a bed, or using a shower jet, rather than doing it with their hands. That may be partly why more women refused to answer.

> **It's possible that women are genuinely less clear than men about what counts as masturbation.**

Other autoerotic activities

Table 6.1 shows the percentage of men and women who had engaged in various autoerotic activities in the previous year.

People who masturbate are more likely to pursue other solitary or media-based sexual activities as well. This may be simply because they have a wider range of things they like to do for sexual arousal and satisfaction. In general, people who haven't had sex with someone else in the last year are also less likely to engage in masturbation or other autoerotic activities. However, people who have had sex with another person at least once but currently have no regular partner are the *most* likely to report autoerotic activities. This suggests there are two kinds of people. Those who are keen on sex tend to have casual sex partners and/or to seek replacement solitary sexual activities if they are not in a relationship. Those who are not as interested in sex don't seem to miss it when they don't have a partner, and they don't seek alternative stimulation.

Table 6.1 Masturbation and related sexual activities in the past year

Sexual activity	Men (%)	Women (%)
Masturbated alone	65	35
Used sex toy	12	14
Had phone sex or rang phone sex line	3	2
Watched X-rated video or film	37	16
Visited Internet sex site on purpose	17	2
Met new partner via Internet chat room	1	<1

Source: Richters et al. 2003, *ANZJPH*, p. 185.

More men than women engaged in autoerotic activities. The single thing women did more of was to use sex toys. By sex toys we mean, for example, a dildo or vibrator. If the respondent asked what counted as a sex toy, the interviewer said that other toys, such as butt plugs or ben-wa balls, were included but not things like feathers, canes or massage oil. We did not specify whether the toy was used for masturbating or in sex with a partner. Women who have masturbated in the past year are five times as likely to have used a sex toy as those who have not, but men who have masturbated are only twice as likely to have used a sex toy. This suggests that much more of the women's use of vibrators and dildos was in masturbation than in partnered sex.

There was no real difference between the number of men and women who said they'd had phone sex or rung a phone sex line. This surprised us, because most of the commercial phone sex services are aimed at male customers. It is possible that women may have included sexy phone calls with lovers, while men regarded only the commercial services as phone sex.

X-rated videos, or non-violent erotica, can be bought legally only from sex shops in the Northern Territory and the Australian Capital Territory. Elsewhere, it's not illegal to buy or possess these videos, only to sell them, so they can be purchased by mail order in all the other Australian states. More than a quarter of the survey respondents have seen an X-rated film in the past year. This suggests that a sizeable minority of Australians are likely to support the continued availability of sexually explicit entertainment and would not welcome the government restricting it further or prohibiting it altogether. Despite the outcry about Internet porn, videos are still seen by far more people. At least, this was true in 2001–02 when the survey was carried out.

People who go to sex websites mostly use them to look at pictures; few people actually meet partners by this method. Less than 1 per cent of people (only three in a thousand women) said they'd met a partner this way in the past year, though it may be that our survey happened just before the number of people doing this increased rapidly. The Internet is probably far more important for people with less common sexual tastes, whether they seek same-sex partners or kinky sex, and whether it's fantasy or to find a real sex partner (see Chapter 7, 'Kinky stuff'). The Internet is also a source of useful information about sexual health and risk-free experimentation with sexual identities and interests. For some young people it can be a huge relief

At 21 Peter is good at making himself come. He started when he was 13. He'd had a spontaneous erection in the shower one morning and it had felt so good when he started washing it he kept doing it, stroking his dick with a soapy hand until all of a sudden this white stuff had come out. He wasn't quite sure what had happened to his body, but worked out that he had just wanked himself off and knew he liked the feeling.

That night Peter tried it when he was in bed. He did the same thing as in the shower, but it wasn't quite the same. Over the next few weeks he experimented with products in the bathroom cupboard before deciding that Vaseline and a tissue worked well.

In that early experimental period Peter knew it was not a cool thing to talk about masturbating to anyone. He started to read things when he got the chance—anything about sex, really—and decided there was nothing wrong with what he was doing even though you were not meant to tell anyone and definitely not let anyone see you doing it. After that Peter became a regular, masturbating at least twice a week.

He bought some old girlie magazines from a garage sale and kept them under his mattress. He also borrowed books with raunchy sex scenes in them from the library. He learnt different ways of making himself come and how to delay his ejaculation. He kept doing it even when he started having sex with girls. The girls certainly liked it that he didn't come straight away, and that was sometimes because he'd masturbated the night before. These days he buys his own glossy magazines, and recently sent away for an X-rated video for the first time—a real high point.

to find others like themselves and to receive non-judgmental advice through websites.

If you can believe what you read in newspapers and magazines, there has recently been a huge increase in the number of Australians using Internet dating services to meet people for relationships. Some of the most popular online dating services for heterosexuals at the moment are RSVP, with more than 350 000 members, and Match.com, with around one million registered Australian users, as well as Matchmaker and Yahoo! Personals. Evidence for the new popularity of online dating includes the 180 per cent increase in traffic on Australian dating sites between March 2002 and February 2004, the publication of *Online Dating for Dummies* and the introduction of a Sydney adult education course on how to 'meet your match online'. However, there has been very little academic research on Net dating, despite some recognition that the Internet may be creating new possibilities for finding love.

Except for the use of sex toys, more men than women enjoyed all of the activities shown in Table 6.1. This may be partly because of the things we asked about. We did not ask about reading sexually explicit novels, which is more common among women, so the questionnaire was slanted towards the kind of things that men are keen on. We considered asking about sexually explicit novels but decided not to because it would have been difficult in a telephone interview to distinguish between a literary novel with a sex scene in it, a sexy historical romance and an erotic story published as erotica such as the Silhouette 'Desire' series. On the other hand, the X-rated classification provided an easy way of identifying films viewed for sexual arousal.

7   kinky stuff

What counts as kinky or even perverted for one person—dressing up in a suspender belt and stockings, say, or spanking—may be a harmless game or sex as usual for another. In this chapter we discuss various sexual practices or games that people can do with a partner, including group sex and various anal erotic practices.

It is perhaps unfair of us to label all the things in this section as 'kinky', as many people regard using their hands to stroke and arouse any part of their partner's body, including the anus, as a normal part of sex, and perhaps do not even think of it as a specific sexual practice.

> **Many people regard using their hands to stroke and arouse any part of their partner's body, including the anus, as a normal part of sex.**

Anal stimulation with the fingers was the most common practice in this list—about one person in six had done this to a partner or had it done to them in the past year (see Table 7.1). These people were also more likely than other respondents to have had multiple sexual partners, or to be gay, lesbian or bisexual, and to have masturbated or done other autoerotic activities. People over fifty and men under twenty were much less likely to have had digital anal stimulation.

Some people would also regard oral–anal stimulation (i.e. licking the anus, also referred to as 'rimming', particularly in the gay community) as a natural extension of oral–genital sex; it was the next most common of these practices, reported by nearly 6 per cent of men and over 3 per cent of women. The other things we asked about in this section were much less common.

Table 7.1 Other sexual activities in the past year among those who had sex

Sexual activity	Men (%)	Women (%)
Role play or dressing up	4	4
B&D, S&M or DS*	2	1
Group sex	2	1
Anal stimulation with fingers**	17	14
Fisting (hand or fist in vagina or rectum)	1	1
Rimming (oral–anal stimulation)	6	3

* Bondage and discipline, sado-masochism or dominance–submission
** Giving or receiving
Source: Richters et al. 2003, ANZJPH, p. 185.

Less than 4 per cent of people engaged in 'role playing or dressing up'. This category—if the interviewer had to clarify it—included playing games, such as 'naughty schoolgirl', or 'captain and cabin boy', or dressing up in fetish gear or (for men) women's clothes. This question was intended as a broad category of sexual games to include activities such as dressing up in sexy lingerie. Such sexual games may contain an element of power-based role playing, but people who play them don't necessarily think of themselves as participating in the S&M scene—that is, in bondage and discipline, sado-masochism, or dominance and submission (see below). Less than 2 per cent of people said they had 'been involved in B&D or S&M'. However, for some people, sexy lingerie, such as corsets, suspender belts and stockings—although regarded as fetish gear by others—may be seen as usual fashion underwear, so they might not have said 'yes' when asked about 'dressing up'.

> **Although magazines occasionally announce epidemics of swinging and group sex in the suburbs, this is apparently more a matter of fantasy.**

Of course, many people who did not say 'yes' to this question may have done things they regard simply as part of sex—such as a bit of spanking for arousal, or playing at threatening a partner with a belt, or tying one partner to the bed—without regarding themselves as people who are 'into' B&D or S&M.

Less than 2 per cent of people, the majority of them male, said they had group sex in the last year. Although magazines occasionally announce epidemics of swinging and group sex in the suburbs, this is apparently more a matter of fantasy or gossip than reality for most people.

Joachim is wise enough to know that not everyone likes to wear leather and be tied up during sex. Now 28, he has a well-developed favourite sexual fantasy. He goes to a fancy-dress party where he meets a woman wearing a leather corset, fishnet stockings and knee-high leather boots. Esmelda is wielding a riding crop that makes a thwack when she strikes the side of her boot with it. To Joachim she is gorgeous, and before long he is literally eating out of her hand. He would do anything she asks.

She takes him to her apartment. Once in the door she orders him onto the floor and makes him crawl into the bedroom. There she hits him with the riding crop on the buttocks and orders him to lie on the bed. She ties him up and then leaves the room. He hears her having a bath. She calls to him that if he behaves himself he might get a 'treat'. When she comes back into the room some time later she is naked except for her boots and riding crop. She stands by the bed lightly stroking him through his leather clothes with the crop, then sits on his face and orders him to lick her. He willingly obeys. When she is satisfied, she leaves him tied up but slowly takes off his pants. After what seems like endless teasing she finally sits down next to him, his erect penis achingly near her vagina. He feels her heat, but cannot move. She strokes his penis lightly with the crop then takes him inside her with one swift motion and in the same action leans back and whacks his feet with the crop. He comes instantly.

Joachim tentatively tried elements of his fantasy on girlfriends, but without success. One thought his liking for leather meant he was actually gay. Another liked to have him spank her, but was increasingly reluctant to return the favour. Then he discovered, through surfing the net, that there was an S&M group in his city. After chatting online for a few weeks he worked up the courage to attend his first fetish party. Reality, he found, was not quite the same as his fantasy.

He learnt from his new friends that you need to take 'safe, sane and consensual' precautions—it's not really sensible to let a complete stranger tie you up and leave the room. He didn't immediately meet someone like Esmelda. There were more women who wanted to be tied up themselves than to tie men up, and some of the women who did enjoy playing dominatrix did it for money. But then he met Anita, and the intense relationship that followed left his fantasy behind.

In the survey we asked about a rather limited list of sexual activities. Other forms of foreplay or sexual scene-setting that we might have explored include tickling, fondling or massage, the use of perfumes and scented oils, candlelit dinners and so on. One reason for avoiding questions about 'romantic' activities or details of pleasure and preference—such as questions about how appealing people find various practices for arousal or for reaching orgasm—is that they can easily become intrusive, flirtatious or sleazy in a phone interview.

Because people's reactions can vary so much, we asked about the less common types of sex in a different section of the questionnaire from the questions about 'what you did the last time you had sex'. That way, if people got offended by the mere mention of the less usual practices, we could simply stop asking the questions and skip to the next section. By the time we asked about rimming (licking the anus) and fisting (inserting the hand or fist into the vagina or rectum—something we did *not* explain to people unfamiliar with the word), 15 per cent of people had stopped answering that set of questions. The rimming question was asked only of people who had experience of oral–genital sex, and the fisting question only of those who had said 'yes' to digital anal stimulation.

There are of course many other much kinkier things we could have asked about. Alfred Kinsey's interviews in the United States in the mid-twentieth century, for example (see Appendix 1: The survey), included questions about sex with animals. He found that about 17 per cent of farm boys, but hardly any urban males, had had sexual contact to orgasm with an animal. However, it is likely that sex with animals, though a constant source of jokes among Australians about New Zealanders, and among the Kiwis about Aussies, is very rare nowadays. If it does happen, it does not seem to cause any ill-effects that bring it to the attention of doctors. Thus there was no reason from the health point of view for us to ask people about it. The same goes for other practices that are probably even rarer, such as necrophilia (sex with corpses), other anal practices such as administering enemas for pleasure, 'water sports' (urine play) or scat (coprophilia or sex play involving faeces). We judged that the risk of offending respondents by the mere mention of these practices was far higher than any possible value in asking the questions.

> **It is likely that sex with animals, though a constant source of jokes among Australians about New Zealanders, and among the Kiwis about Aussies, is rare.**

Most kinky sex of the sort we did ask about is not a health risk, except for the chance of transmitting germs from the bowels to the mouth in anal practices. Even quite way-out sex involving whips and bondage (as long as there is no bleeding) is much less likely to result in people catching HIV or other sexually transmissible infections than is 'normal' intercourse. However, research among gay men has found that men who are into kinky sex are more likely to contract HIV than other gay men. As the kinky things they do are generally less risky than anal intercourse, it seems that it's not the kinky sex itself that is the problem, but the fact that men who are into kinky sex may be more adventurous in general. They may also move in circles (e.g. sex clubs) where a higher proportion of people are infected, making them more likely to come in contact with someone who can pass on the virus.

Traditionally, psychiatrists have seen kinky sexual tastes or activities as 'paraphilias', which are defined as 'disorders that include recurrent, intense sexually arousing fantasies, sexual urges, or behaviors generally involving nonhuman objects, suffering of oneself or partners, or children or other non-consenting partners'. This definition includes exhibitionism (flashing), voyeurism (peeping Tom behaviour), fetishism (preferring sex with inanimate objects), frotteurism (rubbing up against non-consenting people, e.g. in crowded trains) and paedophilia (adults having or desiring sex with young children) as well as sexual masochism, sexual sadism and 'transvestic fetishism' (men dressing up in women's clothes for arousal). Our view as social researchers is rather different, as it is not clear that many of these sexual tastes or activities should be seen as 'disorders' in any way relevant to population health.

Several of the so-called para-philias are socially unacceptable and illegal, not so much because they are sexual but because they involve a non-consenting partner or victim—exhibitionism, voyeur-ism, frotteurism and paedophilia. Fetishism (such as having sex with a blow-up doll) and trans-vestism seem a bit sad or odd to most people, but they are activities without victims. Most people who are into B&D and S&M or other kinds of 'fetish' sex involving role playing, costumes and equipment are not sadistic (in the sense of being cruel) or masochistic (in the sense of wanting to be genuinely abused). Rather they enjoy playing sexual games with other consenting adults, games that involve exaggerating the domi-nating and surrendering elements of sex. In short, the majority of people who indulge in various forms of kinky sex are not obsessed by one particular activity to the exclusion of ordinary sexual practices, but rather people whose sexual repertoire includes a wide range of sexual games, either occasionally for fun or as an ongoing hobby.

Fetishism (such as having sex with a blow-up doll) and trans-vestism seem a bit sad or odd to most people, but they are activities without victims.

8 gay and straight

You may have heard someone at work or at a party or pub say: 'He's gay. I can tell. It's just something about him.' Of course, men sometimes declare a woman is a lesbian just because she does not respond to their expressions of interest. So we don't really know for sure how accurate these people's radar is. Once you start to think about it, defining homosexuality is not as straightforward as it may seem.

A man or woman who is right out there and says, 'I'm gay', is pretty easy to identify—they've done it for you. But what about someone who has sex with someone of the same sex—are they always homosexual? This brings up a whole series of other questions: How do you define sex? Does two women kissing count? Or what about some fondling and intimate touching, but not to orgasm? What if only one person has an orgasm? But what if the person who had the orgasm is happily married and just happened to find themselves in a situation where someone of the same gender touched them in a way that was very arousing? Is that person homosexual?

Sexual identity

There are at least three different ways to think about homosexuality. The first is about *identity*—how people define themselves. Sometimes an 'out' gay man or lesbian dresses and behaves in a certain way that everyone can recognise as 'gay'—such as the stereotypical camp guy on TV, like Jack in the US sitcom *Will and Grace*, or the butch dykes-on-bikes lesbian stereotype.

Gay people often use the term 'out' to describe someone who has 'come out' i.e. announced their homosexual preference to their family and friends. But there are other people who think of themselves as gay, who may be in a same-sex relationship, who don't hide anything and who tick the 'gay/lesbian' box on a questionnaire. Even then, their sexual identity may not be obvious to taxi drivers or people in the pub, perhaps not even to their workmates. This can lead to embarrassing moments at the office party. 'Out' gay people are a statistically small group, with 1.6 per cent of men in our survey identifying as gay and 0.8 per cent of women identifying as lesbian. A further 0.9 per cent of men and 1.4 per cent of women identify as bisexual.

Some bisexuals may be seen by people they meet casually as either gay or straight, depending on how they dress and who they are with. Unless a bisexual person is wearing a 'Bi Pride' button, it can be very hard to tell. Sometimes sexual identity changes during a person's life. For example, a woman who has left a relationship with a man and gone to live with a woman may have described herself as heterosexual in the past but may now regard herself as a lesbian.

Table 8.1 Self-defined sexual identity ('Do you think of yourself as . . .?')

Sexual identity	Men (%)	Women (%)
Heterosexual (straight)	97.4	97.7
Homosexual (gay/lesbian)	1.6	0.8
Bisexual	0.9	1.4

Source: Smith et al. 2003, *ANZJPH*, p. 141.

Sexual attraction

The second way to think about homosexuality is about *attraction*—whether a man or woman is attracted to someone of the same sex, regardless of whether they act upon this feeling. Obviously there are different levels of intensity of attraction, but overall, 7 per cent of men and 13 per cent of women have been attracted at least once to someone of the same sex. Exclusive same-sex attraction is much less common (0.6 per cent men, 0.2 per cent women). The US researcher Alfred Kinsey thought of same-sex attraction with no sexual interest in the opposite sex as one end of a continuum of sexual interest. However, some people are highly sexually interested in both men and women, and some

Unless a bisexual person is wearing a 'Bi Pride' button, it can be very hard to tell.

are sexually attracted to no one (0.2 per cent men, 0.6 per cent women), so perhaps it is better to think in terms of two separate spectrums of sexual attraction, one for men and one for women.

For some people, sexual attractiveness is not primarily about gender. They find things attractive in both men and women—perhaps body type, or sense of humour, or musical interests, or a way-out sexual style. This can seem puzzling to 'monosexuals' (those who fancy only people of one sex), whether they're exclusive homosexuals who have tried and failed to find opposite-sex people sexy, or straight people who think it 'natural' to find lots of opposite-sex people of about the right age attractive.

Table 8.2 Lifetime sexual attraction to same and opposite sex

Sexual attraction	Men (%)	Women (%)
Only to opposite sex	92.9	86.5
More often to opposite sex	4.5	11.0
About equally often to both sexes	0.6	1.0
Mostly to same sex	1.1	0.6
Only to same sex	0.6	0.2
No one	0.2	0.6

Source: Smith et al. 2003, *ANZJPH*, p. 141.

Sexual experience

The third way to think about homosexuality is to use *sexual experience* as the defining factor. This means having had some form of sexual experience with someone of the same sex as you. About 6 per cent of men and 9 per cent of women have had at least some sexual contact with a person of the same sex in their lives. However, less than 2 per cent of men and women had sex with a same-sex partner in the past year.

Table 8.3 Lifetime sexual experience with same and opposite sex

Sexual experience	Men (%)	Women (%)
Only with opposite sex	90.7	88.3
More often with opposite sex	4.0	7.5
About equally often with both sexes	0.4	0.5
Mostly with same sex	1.0	0.4
Only with same sex	0.6	0.1
No one	3.3	3.1

Source: Smith et al. 2003, *ANZJPH*, p. 141.

So who's straight, who's gay?

Some same-sex attraction or experience was reported by 9 per cent of men and 15 per cent of women. Hardly anyone (no men and only a few women) identifies as bisexual or gay without having some same-sex attraction or experience. For most people, most of the time, attraction, experience and identity correspond—the majority of heterosexuals have sex with opposite-sex partners, most gay men have sex with men, most lesbians have sex with women and most bisexuals have sex with both men and women. However, you cannot assume that someone who identifies as gay or lesbian has never had straight sex—60 per cent of gay men have had sex with a woman, and 82 per cent of lesbians have had sex with a man. Social pressure to conform to the heterosexual norm can be very strong.

People seem, not surprisingly, to be happiest when their sexual attraction, experience and identity correspond. Indeed, men who find other men attractive but have never acted on that attraction are more likely to be anxious and miserable than other men. Among women, those who had any same-sex experience or attraction were more likely to feel sad or anxious.

Tables 8.4 and 8.5 show that there are fewer gays and lesbians than there are heterosexuals with same-sex experience. However, most heterosexuals with same-sex experience have only had one same-sex partner (see Chapter 4, 'How many partners').

Table 8.4 Relationship between current sexual identity and lifetime sexual attraction and experience for men

	Heterosexual	Homosexual (gay)	Bisexual	Total
Attracted only to females; experience only with females	91.4 %	0.0%	0.0%	91.4%
Attracted only to females; some experience with males	1.7%	0.0%	<0.1%	1.7%
Some attraction to males; experience only with females	2.5%	<0.1%	<0.1%	2.5%
Some attraction to males; some experience with males	2.0%	1.6%	0.8%	4.4%
Total	97.4%	1.6%	0.9%	100.0%

Source: Smith et al. 2003, *ANZJPH*, p. 141.

Table 8.5 Relationship between current sexual identity and lifetime sexual attraction and experience for women

	Heterosexual	Homosexual (lesbian)	Bisexual	Total
Attracted only to males; experience only with males	84.8%	0.0%	0.0%	84.9%
Attracted only to males; some experience with females	1.9%	0.0%	0.0%	1.9%
Some attraction to females; experience only with males	6.2%	0.0%	0.1%	6.3%
Some attraction to females; some experience with females	4.7%	0.8%	1.3%	6.9%
Total	97.7%	0.8%	1.4%	100.0%

Source: Smith et al. 2003, *ANZJPH*, p. 141.

The men and women most likely to have same-sex experience have tertiary education and white-collar or professional jobs. Men and women who speak a language other than English at home, men living in remote or regional places and men in blue-collar occupations are the least likely to have any same-sex experience.

Almost all of the men who have had some same-sex experience but identify as heterosexual have had sex with only one other male. Nearly a quarter of these same-sex experiences happened when they were fifteen or younger. The same proportion of gay men had their first same-sex experience when they were under sixteen, so it seems that experimenting with sex with another boy does not make a boy more likely to grow up gay.

The men and women most likely to have same-sex experience have tertiary education and white-collar or professional jobs.

Similarly, almost all of the women who identify as heterosexual but have some same-sex experience had sex with only one other female. Only 16 per cent of heterosexual women with same-sex experience had it for the first time when they were under sixteen, and nearly half were 21 or older. Lesbian women were even older on average when they first had sex with a woman—only 9 per cent were under sixteen, and more than half were over 21.

There is some evidence that young men nowadays who see themselves as heterosexual are less likely to have had any same-sex contact than men in their fathers' or grandfathers' generation. One reason may be that with the rise in contraceptive use and acceptance of sex between adolescents, it is easier for young men to have sex with girlfriends. At the same time, people are much more conscious of homosexuality. Boys tend to be hyper-aware of anything that might make other kids accuse them of homosexuality. 'Poofter' and 'gay' are used as terms of abuse in primary school playgrounds, even before kids know what they mean. But boys soon work out that certain sexual practices—any touching of another male's penis included—will brand them as gay. A study of university students in Germany, done in 1970 and repeated in 1990, found a large drop between the two surveys in the number of young men who did not identify as gay but reported same-sex activity. The authors suggested that boys in the 1990s could not do anything with another boy without labelling themselves as gay.

The picture that emerges is that homosexuality is better known nowadays than thirty or forty years ago and more acceptable among younger people.

In our survey, the percentage of men who had any sexual experience with another male in their lifetime was the same for men in their twenties, thirties, forties and fifties. Not many men have had some sexual experience with a male despite not being sexually attracted to males (see the second row of figures in Table 8.4), but this is much more common for men over forty than for younger men.

The situation appears to be different for women. Younger women are more likely than older women to have had sex with another female, and same-sex experience among women who are not sexually attracted to females is more common among women in their twenties and less so among older age groups, especially the over-fifties.

The picture that emerges is that homosexuality is better known nowadays than thirty or forty years ago and more acceptable among younger people. However, partly as a result of that greater awareness, it is harder for boys today to 'mess around' with each other without thinking of themselves as gay. At the same time, same-sex activity does not seem to lead to girls being regarded as lesbians, and young women are much more likely than their mothers to have experimented with sex with another girl.

Gavin came out to his parents when he left school. Although they were a bit shocked, they coped and have come to accept him as he is. After a few years of being 'out', Gavin felt part of the gay community in the city. Some of his friends told him about the different places you can go to meet other gay men, depending on what you are looking for. So sometimes Gavin would meet guys in bars or in clubs, but if he was just looking for sex then he would usually go to a sex venue.

While some of his gay friends aren't into the casual sex scene, Gavin really likes it that everyone is there to have sex, so you can hook up with a guy and not have to get to know him first. And although Gavin could also do this at outdoor beats, he usually prefers being somewhere that feels safer and has a friendlier atmosphere. He also likes the fact that you can have sex with more than one man in a night, and can usually have the kind of sex you want, maybe just a blow job or anal sex as well.

Gavin has had sex with dozens of guys in the past few months and has made some new friends along the way. He has even met his first true love in the back room of a sex venue!

Do people tell the truth about homosexuality?

One way to tell whether a question in a survey is very sensitive is to look at how many people refuse to answer it. The refusal rates for these questions about homosexuality—a good indicator of people's discomfort—were about 0.1 per cent, much lower than for masturbation (2 per cent men, 5 per cent women) or income (5 per cent overall). It is possible that people 'forget' to report early experiences that do not fit with their current sexual identity—for example a straight, married man may not tell our interviewer about the time in his teens when he was sucked off by a truck driver who gave him a lift. But this would not make any difference to the reported rates of gay, lesbian or bisexual identity. Unless gay people are much more likely to refuse to be interviewed—and we have no evidence that this is the case—our estimates are likely to be accurate.

So what percentage of the population is gay?

It is too simple to say '10 per cent of the population is gay', but it is true that at least 10 per cent of the population is a little bit gay-ish, either in experience or attraction or both. Although gay men and lesbians often say they were aware of the direction of their sexual feelings from a very early age, many teenagers

Michelle was confused. She got top marks in her uni courses, had lots of friends and her parents loved her, but she just wasn't sure whether she liked guys or girls sexually. The trouble was, there was a gorgeous girl called Lisa in one of her classes. She had a strong face with a beautiful smile, short cropped blond hair and ultra-smooth slightly olive skin. She wore tops that showed just a hint of deep cleavage and Michelle found herself wondering what they would feel like if she cupped them in her hands. Last night she held her own breasts and fantasised that they were Lisa's while she masturbated.

Michelle was not a virgin and she had enjoyed sex with boys. She couldn't work out why she was so attracted to Lisa. She'd never had any kind of sex with a woman before. She didn't count the kiss she shared with Melinda at a party. It was almost a dare and both of them had been so nervous they never talked about it again. It just wasn't the same. It might have been the way Lisa looked at her, as if she wanted her, but Michelle thought she might be imagining that. She wouldn't know what to do if Lisa asked her out or something.

A week later Michelle bumped into Lisa leaving a lecture hall just before lunch. Lisa asked her if she wanted to have lunch together, so they did. Michelle didn't know what to say and just looked a little dumbstruck. Then Lisa asked her, a bit hesitantly, whether she was okay: 'Are you all right? You look like you've just met a spunky boy—you're not gay are you? Some gay girls see the short hair and think I am too.'

are unsure about their sexuality. Schoolteachers need to remember that about three kids in the average class may not feel themselves to be exclusively heterosexual. For adolescents with little practical experience of sex, grappling with uncertain sexuality can be stressful. This can be exacerbated by peer pressure to conform to limited stereotypes of acceptable gender behaviour—kids who are perceived to be 'different' can be given a hard time.

When questions about homosexuality have been asked in rigorous scientific sexual behaviour surveys in the United Kingdom and the United States, results similar to those in Australia have been found. In the United States in 1992, 3 per cent of men and 1 per cent of women identified as homosexual or bisexual. Same-sex contact in their lifetime was reported by 9 per cent of men and 4 per cent of women, and same-sex attraction by 6 per cent of men and 4 per cent of women. In the UK in 1991, same-sex experience was reported by 5 per cent of men and 3 per cent of women, and same-sex attraction by 10 per cent of men and 5 per cent of women. In the 2000 follow-up study, 5 per cent of men and women reported having had at least one same-sex experience.

These figures are not very different from ours. The main difference is that more Australian women than men report same-sex attraction and experience. Interestingly, only a third of the women who reported both same-sex attraction and experience identified as lesbian or bisexual; the rest identified as heterosexual. It seems that in Australian society it is easier for women than for men to acknowledge and act on same-sex desires, while retaining a primarily straight identity.

Some readers, especially those who live in the centre of the larger cities, might have expected the survey to report a higher proportion of people identifying as gay. One reason why the percentage may strike them as low is the tendency for gay people to migrate to large cities, and often to certain suburbs. This is sometimes because small communities can be intolerant of homosexual behaviour and, not surprisingly, many gay people like to meet and socialise with other gay people. This creates something of a cluster effect where the percentage of people who identify as gay or engage in homosexual behaviour is much higher than in other parts of the country.

For adolescents with little practical experience of sex, grappling with uncertain sexuality can be stressful.

9 domestic bliss

In the survey our definition of a 'regular relationship' was broad, including any sexual relationship that the respondent expected would continue, in the sense that they would have sex together again. At any one time, the majority of people (75 per cent) are in regular heterosexual relationships. The remaining 25 per cent, then, includes gay men and lesbians, young people who are not yet ready to pair up with anyone, people who stay single (some of whom have sex with casual partners) and older people who are widowed, divorced or separated (some of whom are not looking for a new partner), as well as people who are seeking a partner. No wonder people who are 'on the market' again after a break-up get the impression that everyone else is part of a couple and that there are very few potential partners, especially in the older age groups. Of the people in regular heterosexual relationships, 83 per cent are living together, and about half the relationships have lasted more than ten years.

Unlike women and straight men, only about half the gay and bisexual men are in regular relationships. As we've seen, gay men are more likely to have sex with many different partners.

About half the people in the survey are legally married (see Table 9.1). A few of the divorced and separated people, as well as many of the never married, are in regular relationships. Indeed, a few of the legally married people may be living with someone other than the person they are married to.

> **Unlike women and straight men, only about half the gay and bisexual men are in regular relationships.**

Table 9.1 Legal marital status

	Men (%)	Women (%)
Married	50	54
Divorced	7	8
Separated	3	4
Widowed	1	1
Never married	40	33

Source: Data from ASHR.

Table 9.2 Age differences in regular heterosexual relationships

Age of partner relative to respondent	Men (%)	Women (%)
More than 5 years younger	21	4
1 to 5 years younger	52	19
Same age	11	14
1 to 5 years older	13	47
More than 5 years older	3	16

Source: Rissel et al. 2003, *ANZJPH*, p. 126.

It is still common that men tend to have slightly younger women as partners, and women slightly older men, but there are exceptions. Table 9.2 shows, for example, that 3 per cent of men have partners more than five years older than themselves, and 4 per cent of women have partners more than five years younger.

Almost universally, both men and women expect themselves and their partners not to have sex with other people (see Chapter 10, 'Is your partner cheating on you?').

Satisfaction with relationships

Most people seem to be very happy in their regular relationships. In fact, 87 per cent of men and 79 per cent of women said their relationship was 'very' or 'extremely' emotionally satisfying. Only 2 per cent of men and 5 per cent of women said their relationship was not at all satisfying, or only slightly. English speakers, especially men, were more likely than those speaking other languages to say their relationship was extremely emotionally satisfying.

People seemed to be happiest when their relationships had lasted one to five years. Women were likely to be extremely happy with new relationships, while men were not. Figure 9.1

shows that men are more likely than women to be extremely emotionally satisfied with their relationship when it has lasted more than a year, but women are more enthusiastic than men about new relationships. Indeed, women's emotional satisfaction drops in the second year at the same time that men's rises.

Men's lack of keenness in the early months of a relationship may explain women's frequent complaint that men are 'commitment-phobic'. It has been suggested that men do not relate to women as individuals on a person-to-person level, rather than as exchangeable companions to enjoy oneself with, except in committed relationships. It seems that it takes men longer to feel safe enough to open up emotionally and enjoy intimacy. They fear self-revelation and 'getting in deep', but once they've done so, they appear to be less likely to be emotionally disappointed with the relationship later on.

Women were likely to be extremely happy with new relationships, while men were not.

There was a clear pattern that the more often people (both men and women) had sex, the more likely they were to be extremely emotionally satisfied with their regular relationship. People who had sexual difficulties (see Chapter 13, 'Sexual difficulties') were less likely to have extremely satisfying

Figure 9.1 People who said their regular heterosexual relationship was extremely emotionally satisfying

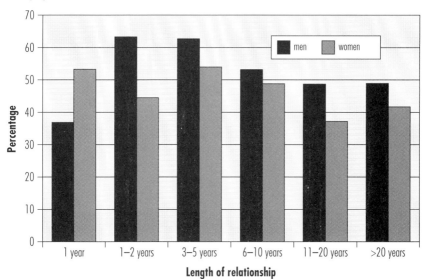

Source: Richters et al. 2003, *ANZJPH*, p. 175.

relationships. Of course we can't tell whether people have more sex because their relationships are happy, or whether having good sex makes them get on better in other ways. Probably both are true.

Women who identified as bisexual were less likely to find their regular relationship with a man emotionally satisfying. However, they were just as likely as heterosexual women to enjoy the sex they had with their male partners (see below). This suggests that for women there is a link between being emotionally dissatisfied with relationships with men and identifying as bisexual rather than straight. It is not just a matter of being sexually attracted to women.

Physical pleasure in sex

It seems that Australians like sex—90 per cent of men and 79 per cent of women said the sex in their regular relationship was 'very' or 'extremely' pleasurable. But overall, sex is more fun for men than women. Hardly any men—just over 1 per cent—say sex is slightly or not at all pleasurable, but 5 per cent of women say this.

The youngest men are most enthusiastic about sex if they are having any—63 per cent of those under twenty say the sex

Men have the best sex in relationships that have lasted one to five years, whereas women enjoy the sex best in new relationships.

in their relationship is extremely pleasurable, and the rate falls with age to 42 per cent of men in their fifties. Only 33 per cent of women under twenty say that the sex in their relationship is extremely pleasurable. Among women, the age group most likely to find sex extremely pleasurable (48 per cent) are those in their twenties. The rate then falls with age to 27 per cent of women in their fifties.

English speakers, both men and women, are much more likely to say sex is extremely pleasurable than those who speak other languages. This may be because it is not culturally appropriate for people from some backgrounds to sound so enthusiastic about sex.

Men have the best sex in relationships that have lasted one to five years, whereas women enjoy the sex best in new relationships (see Figure 9.2). Both men and women are less excited about the physical pleasure of the sex in relationships of over twenty years, when they are older. Women's enthusiasm for the sex in new relationships mirrors their emotional satisfaction. This throws a new light on women's complaints that men avoid commitment. Is it because women are so full-on early in a relationship that men are uncomfortable? Or do men often commence relationships with women they do not really like, just to get sex, and then need to extricate themselves?

Figure 9.2 People who said the sex in their regular heterosexual relationship was extremely physically pleasurable

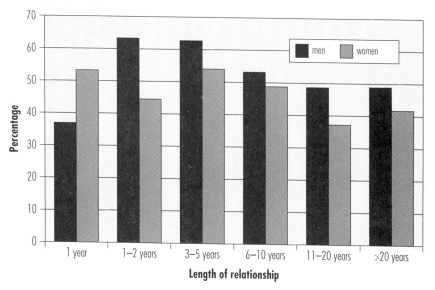

Source: Richters et al. 2003, *ANZJPH*, p. 174.

The few bisexual men in relationships with women seemed less happy with the sex they had with their partners than straight men were, but the bisexual women (and indeed the very few lesbians in relationships with men) seemed to enjoy sex with their male partners just as much (or as little) as straight women.

Perhaps not surprisingly, the more often people had sex with their regular partners the more likely they were to say it was extremely good.

Roger wished he was more like his mate Steve. Steve was the same age—29—but had now been married to the lovely Caroline for three years. Every time he saw them together they were all over each other, holding hands, giving little kisses, and standing or sitting so close you'd think they were stuck together. They had a lot in common and it seemed they really understood each other. And from what Steve said, in bed they went at it like rabbits. The sex was good and so was the relationship—there had to be some chemistry there.

Roger firmly believed in that whole chemistry thing, that you had to get on together sexually or a relationship would never last. That was pretty well how he operated when he was out trying to meet women. He'd always go for the sexiest one, the one with shapely legs, or full breasts, or who turned him on in some way. He wasn't in bad shape himself. He spoke softly and dressed well, so he felt confident his advances would at least have a chance. But things generally didn't last too well. His longest relationship had been 14 months.

He knew at some level it wasn't really the woman's fault. After all, it was usually him that ended it. He'd meet someone, be very attentive, send flowers and do that sort of thing, just like it said in the magazines, and then after a few dates (or sometimes straight away) they would have sex. The first time he usually enjoyed it heaps. Roger really liked sex, he was pretty adventurous in bed and the woman usually enjoyed it too. But after a few months or so, something just seemed to go wrong. She would ask him questions about himself and think he was being secretive when he said he didn't know the answers. He sort of lost interest, and blamed the woman or their lack of chemistry together for it not working out. Sometimes it was difficult breaking up if the woman had started to think the relationship might be getting serious.

is your partner cheating on you?

As we saw in Chapter 5, 'Attitudes towards sex', most Australians hold firmly to the idea that being in a committed relationship (including but not only marriage) means that it is wrong to have sex with someone else—78 per cent of both men and women think it is 'always wrong' to have an affair. This is reflected in their statements that they considered their own male–female relationship to be sexually exclusive: 96 per cent of men and women said they expected their partner not to have sex with anyone else, and 94 per cent of men and 97 per cent of women said they themselves expected not to have sex with anyone other than their partner. It is notable that men and women are equally likely to expect sexual fidelity from their partners, but men are slightly less likely to apply the rule to their own behaviour.

Who counts as a 'sexual partner'?

In the questionnaire (see Appendix 3) we asked each person how many men or women they had had intercourse with. Then we asked whether there were any people they had had oral sex (but not intercourse) with and lastly whether there was anyone else they had other kinds of sexual contact with 'that involved stimulating the penis or vaginal area' (this would include 'manual sex' or petting). These were added together to get the total number of male and female partners for each respondent. However, when we asked separately about sexual experience with men and women, we were much more generous in our definition, introducing the question with these words: 'In the next question when we say "sexual experience" we mean any kind of contact with another person that you felt was sexual. It could be kissing or touching, or intercourse, or any form of sex.' The result was that more people said they'd had some sexual experience. Clearly some people have had experiences that they consider to be sexual, but which didn't include intercourse or other kinds of genital stimulation. This means that the figures in this chapter for numbers of same-sex partners do not quite match the figures given in Chapter 8 ('Gay and straight') for people who have had same-sex experiences.

Table 10.1 Ages of people expecting not to have sex with anyone other than their opposite-sex regular partner

Age group	Men (%)	Women (%)
16–19	90	94
20–29	92	97
30–39	97	99
40–49	95	99
50–59	96	98
Total	94	97

Source: Rissel et al. 2003b, ANZJPH, p. 128.

Table 10.2 Sexual identity of people expecting not to have sex with anyone other than their opposite-sex regular partner

Sexual identity	Men (%)	Women (%)
Heterosexual	95	98
Bisexual	43	78
Total	94	97

Very few gay men and lesbians were in regular relationships with an opposite-sex partner, so they have not been included.

Source: Rissel et al. 2003b, ANZJPH, p. 128.

Asked whether they had discussed the question of having sex with someone else with their partner, 57 per cent of men and 73 per cent of women said they had discussed it and agreed with their partner. This large difference between men's and women's replies indicates that women are far more likely than men to believe they have agreed with their partner about the rules in the relationship. There seem to be some conversations women have had that men have not 'heard'. Only a few people (4 per cent) who had discussed their expectations had failed to agree (or at least that was the respondent's perception).

Many people expected that they and their partner would not have sex with anyone else, but they had not discussed it explicitly. This suggests people see this as a natural implication of being in a regular relationship, or perhaps as an understood, though unstated, implication of living together or marriage. In a traditional culture with rules accepted by everyone about sex before or outside of marriage, it may not be necessary for people to discuss such a matter explicitly. In some cultures—and among some people in Australia—a certain amount of sexual freedom for men is regarded as natural, even when those men are married or in a regular relationship. Visiting sex workers may be common and accepted (see Chapter 15, 'Paying for sex'). But in a pluralist society like Australia it would seem prudent for couples to talk to each other about what they expect. Otherwise one partner may do something that he or she thinks of as just 'playing around' but the other partner sees as signalling the end of the relationship: 'How could he possibly do that if he still loves me?'.

Presumably, many people in relationships do not 'discuss explicitly' and agree about whether they can have sex with anyone else because for them the very meaning of a 'committed' relationship is that it is one-to-one. At weddings, people tease the couple and remind them that their time for playing around is over—this means having sex with only one person for the rest of their lives! When the scandal of US President Bill Clinton's affair with Monica Lewinsky was in the news, most people just assumed that if Clinton had had sex with Lewinsky he was unfaithful to his wife—that's what marriage means to most people. Yet for all we know the Clintons may have had an agreement such as, 'It's okay if you play around as long as it's not serious and no one knows about it', or 'It's all right as long as there's no intercourse'. Of course, even if that were the case, for the Clintons to admit such a thing publicly would not have been acceptable to the conservative Christian groups in the United States.

Monogamy and fidelity

People often refer to having only one regular, committed partner at a time as 'monogamy'. They often also use the word to mean not having sex with anyone else (although these are not necessarily quite the same thing). And neither meaning is the same as the dictionary definition of the word, which is 'marriage of one woman with one man' (in contrast to polygamy) or 'the practice of marrying only once during life' (*Macquarie Dictionary: Second edition*, 1991). Because of the possible confusion surrounding

For many people, sex with someone else just *is* infidelity and a threat to the relationship.

this, we have not used the terms 'monogamy' or 'monogamous'.

Another term that is used in this context is 'fidelity'. For many people, sex with someone else just *is* infidelity and a threat to the relationship, however careful the straying partner is about avoiding infection or pregnancy. Other people talk about this and come to an agreement about whether sex with anyone else is allowed in the relationship and if so under what conditions. This is discussed further in Chapter 16, 'Sexually transmitted infections and safe sex'. Fidelity need not be only about sex. For some people, there are worse ways of being unfaithful—such as taking money from a joint savings account meant for a deposit on a house to buy a power boat or an overseas trip; or letting the partner down with promises such as picking up the children from child care; or not supporting the partner through a life crisis such as illness or losing their job. This notion of fidelity is about mutual caring and commitment to the couple's joint aims and responsibilities rather than about sexual exclusivity.

Among respondents who expect exclusivity from themselves and their partners, 68 per cent have discussed this. Similarly among those who do not expect exclusivity from themselves or their partners, 70 per cent have discussed this. But among people who have a mixed response on exclusivity—those who expected their partner to sleep around but not to do it them-selves, or vice versa—only about half had discussed the issue. This suggests that the topic is often not discussed precisely because it is so threatening. Someone (more often but not always a woman) who places a high value on sexual exclusiv-ity, and who wants to maintain their relationship with their partner, may well choose not to raise the issue in case the answer is 'Look, I may well have sex with other people and I don't mind if you do too'. This would lead to a complete clash between two strongly held beliefs—not wanting to change their view of infidelity, but also not wanting to leave their partner. In this case it might be better not to ask.

People who expect exclusivity from themselves and their partner are more likely to agree when they have their discussion than people who don't expect it from either partner. Where the expectations are different for the two partners, the couple are much less likely to agree. It appears that some 'open' relation-ships contain one partner who does not want this arrangement. This also highlights the possible ambiguity of the word 'expect'— you might expect your partner not to have sex with anyone else in the sense of thinking it morally wrong if he or she were to do so, but in fact expect (i.e. think it likely) that he or she will.

How many people do play around?

Among people who have been in a regular relationship with an opposite-sex partner for 12 months or more, 5 per cent of men and 3 per cent of women have had sex with someone else in the past year. People who have had sex with someone other than their regular partner are likely to be young (mostly under 30), are more likely to be bisexual and are less likely to be married. Those who are legally separated or divorced are more likely to have had sex outside their current regular relationship than those who are widowed or have never married. (One might speculate that this sort of behaviour is what led to the break-up of their marriage.) Sex outside a regular relationship is much more common among gay men than among heterosexuals. (This is discussed further in Chapter 16, 'Sexually transmitted infections and safe sex').

Among both men and women who currently expect themselves not to have sex with anyone else, only around 2 per cent have had sex with someone other than their regular partner in the past year. It's possible that since this happened they have changed their minds about what they expect to do in the future.

All the signs were bad. Richard had started working back late, had a shower when he got home late at night, was often tired and didn't feel like having sex as often as he used to. Susan, his wife of 19 years, knew it couldn't be anyone at work, as all the women in his office were just far too young for this mid-forties man—he could almost be their father.

When they'd first got married they'd talked about being faithful to each other and how they were not interested in an 'open' relationship. Had all that suddenly changed? Susan, remembering a video they'd seen recently of the swinging seventies, felt sick at the thought of some sort of partner-swapping arrangement with their close friends. Sure, sex with Richard wasn't always screaming with ecstatic excitement, but they were comfortable with each other's bodies. That had to count for something.

That night when he came home at 11 p.m. she was waiting for him. First thing she did was get up close and smell him, searching for the smell of sex or perfume. He had his familiar odour of sweat and a hint of the after-shave he always wore.

Richard backed away, knowing that he was going to have to tell her what was going on. All he was doing was overtime—helping the stock-take guys move things around after hours. He was trying to put away some extra money so he could surprise her for their twentieth wedding anniversary with a nice romantic holiday away. So much for surprise!

Sex outside the relationship is much more common among the small group of people who expect it—about 60 per cent of people who do not expect sexual exclusivity of themselves have had sex with someone else in the past year. People's expectations are a reasonably good guide to what they actually do.

So, in short, if you've talked about this with your partner, and you've both agreed that he or she won't have sex with anyone else, it's a reasonable bet that your partner isn't cheating on you.

11 getting pregnant

For many women there comes a time when they deliberately stop using contraception because they want to have a baby. Other pregnancies happen when they were not intended—but not all these pregnancies are unwanted. Sometimes pregnancy is the result of a one-night stand (clearly without a condom!) or it might even be the first time a teenager has sex. Some women have difficulty getting pregnant and they and their partners need to seek medical assistance. For many people, pregnancy and childbirth are natural and straightforward, but not everyone's experience is the same.

Though very few women in the survey regard themselves as infertile, one woman in six (16 per cent) had some difficulty getting pregnant, and half of these women had treatment. Overall, three-quarters of women who have had intercourse have been pregnant at least once (see Table 11.1). The age at which women first became pregnant ranged from fourteen to 43.

Table 11.1 Fertility and pregnancy among women who have ever had intercourse

	Women (%)
Ever been pregnant	76
Ever used emergency contraception	19
Ever had problems getting pregnant	16
Ever had treatment to help getting pregnant	8

Source: Smith et al. 2003, ANZJPH, p. 206.

Of women who have been pregnant most have delivered a live baby (see Table 11.2). This amounts to 70 per cent of all women. The most babies any woman in the survey has had is 11. One woman in three had a miscarriage. Of these, most have only ever had one miscarriage, but some had two, three or more—one woman had fifteen miscarriages. Few women had stillbirths, but even this distressing experience can happen more than once—the maximum in the survey was four stillbirths.

The most babies any woman in the survey has had is 11.

Table 11.2 Pregnancy outcomes among women who have ever been pregnant

	Women (%)
Ever had a live birth	92
Ever had a miscarriage	33
Ever had a stillbirth	3
Ever had a termination of pregnancy (abortion)	23
Ever had a child who was given up for adoption	1

Source: Smith et al. 2003, *ANZJPH*, p. 206.

Table 11.3 Outcomes of the 21 060 pregnancies reported to the survey

	Pregnancies (%)
Live birth	72
Miscarriage	17
Stillbirth	1
Termination	10

Source: Smith et al. 2003, *ANZJPH*, p. 208.

Women now in their twenties are more likely to regard themselves as too young to be mothers.

Almost a quarter of women in the survey who had been pregnant had a termination of pregnancy (abortion). The number of abortions reported by any one woman ranges from one to twelve, but three-quarters of the women who experienced abortion had only one and few had three or more. Women in their fifties are less likely to have had an abortion, because their sexually active lives commenced in the 1960s when abortion was still illegal and therefore risky (or very expensive), stigmatised and difficult to obtain. Women in their twenties are more likely to have had an abortion (34 per cent) than those in their thirties (24 per cent). This probably reflects the current tendency to delay childbearing until the thirties—women now in their twenties are more likely to regard themselves as too young to be mothers, or not yet in a stable relationship or job, than was the case twenty years ago. However, only about 10 per cent of pregnancies result in a termination (see Table 11.3). Since abortion became effectively legal and parenting payments have been available to single mothers, very few women have chosen to go through with an unwanted pregnancy and give up the baby for adoption. Only ninety new babies were given up for adoption during 1997–98 compared with the peak of nearly 10 000 babies given up in 1971–72.

Teenage pregnancy

Fewer women are having children in their teens today than forty years ago. Figure 11.1 shows that 23 per cent of women now in their fifties became pregnant while they were teenagers in the late 1950s and 60s, but those now in their twenties were less likely to have done so. Teenage pregnancy has been declining since the 1970s, but it is still much higher in Australia than in some European countries—though less of a problem here than in the United Kingdom or the United States, which has the developed world's highest rates of teenage pregnancy. In countries where sexual activity between teenagers is accepted, openness and supportive attitudes do not lead to teenagers having more sex or taking more risks. Sex education in countries with lower teenage pregnancy rates emphasises responsibility, pregnancy prevention and knowledge about HIV and other sexually transmissible diseases. It also helps if parenthood is explicitly regarded as something you do when you become an independent adult, and teenagers are assisted to become independent. In the United States, sexuality education programs often promote abstinence only. As American teenagers are surrounded by sex in the media, they receive very conflicting messages from adults.

> **Sex education in countries with lower teenage pregnancy rates emphasises responsibility, pregnancy prevention and knowledge about HIV and other sexually transmissible diseases.**

Figure 11.1 Women pregnant for the first time before age 20

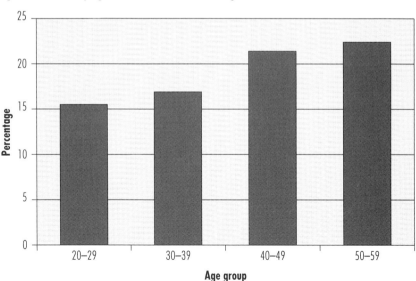

Source: Smith et al. 2003, ANZJPH, pp. 204–9.

In Australia, teenagers from well-off suburbs and with more education are less likely to have babies before they turn twenty. This is partly because—as we saw in Chapter 1, 'First times'—

people who finish school and go to university tend to start having sex later than those who leave school early and move into the adult world of work or unemployment. Also the educated adolescents are more likely to use contraception, including emergency contraception. Furthermore, if a better educated young woman does fall pregnant she is more likely to have an abortion than to go through with the pregnancy. Nowadays most teenagers who give birth keep the baby and raise it themselves, unless the social services intervene to protect the baby's safety. This is rare, but it can happen (and not only to young mothers), for example if the mother is a continuing heavy user of drugs such as heroin.

In our culture, teenage pregnancy is generally regarded as a bad thing, although biologically speaking, there is no reason for a woman not to give birth once she is physically mature, over about sixteen. The reasons are social. Women who have babies when they are under twenty are more likely to leave full-time education, be unemployed and be single mothers. Now that more and more women are delaying child-bearing until their education is complete and they are financially established and in a stable relationship, many are not having their first child until their thirties or even their early forties. This is reflected in the difficulties that many women now have in getting pregnant—they start trying well after the age when they are most fertile. Women who have their first babies in their thirties or forties are also more likely to have complications that require interventions, such as caesarean section.

Perhaps it is time for Australia to look at ways of supporting instead of discouraging young parents so that this trend of late childbearing does not continue indefinitely. It is understandable that each woman making a decision about her own fertility perceives the economic and social benefits of having children later, when she is more established in her work, or she and her partner have bought a house. But the effect at the community level is that first-time parents are getting older and older, and more and more would-be parents need to resort to IVF and other forms of assisted conception to have a child— and ten-year-olds have middle-aged parents. So it is at the community level that we need to give more support to parents. With more help for young parents, having a child need not be such a daunting undertaking that only someone over 35 can face it.

Margaret and Tony agreed they wanted children, but they wanted to establish themselves first, so when the time was right they could really be involved with the kids. Margaret didn't want to have to work full time while the kids were small. She and Tony were hard workers and enjoyed their work, but they also liked good holidays overseas. They saved for a deposit on a house when prices weren't completely astronomical, but they also knew that when they had kids they'd need a bigger place.

Margaret was 36 by the time they realised they couldn't wait any longer. She stopped taking the pill and started to watch her menstrual cycle for the fertile period. That was the part Tony liked the most—feeling like a prize stud with Margaret waiting for it.

Unfortunately she didn't just fall pregnant. After 18 months they both had fertility tests to see if there was a biological reason they couldn't get pregnant. There wasn't. They kept trying, and thought about whether they could afford the cost of the IVF program. From what their friends had told them, it was emotionally stressful, with hormones all over the place, lots of injections, and no guarantee of success. Getting pregnant was not meant to be like that.

They kept trying for a natural pregnancy for another year. Tony stopped enjoying sex as much as it was almost getting to be some kind of chore. They decided to stop focusing on it for a while, then started to resign themselves to the possibility that they might not be able to have children. They went on holiday to a peaceful Pacific island and had a great time. Then four months later, Margaret found she was pregnant. She said nothing at work until it was quite obvious. She couldn't bear the thought of losing it and having to tell everyone.

12 not getting pregnant

Some of the readers of this book will remember the days when GPs had little or no training in contraception. Indeed, some of them actively disapproved of it. To get informed and helpful family planning care then, you needed to go to a Family Planning Association clinic or a doctor who specialised in 'women's matters', especially if you were unmarried. Today most GPs offer well-informed assistance with contraception. This is reflected in our survey results. Of the few women who said they did not use contraception even though they were having sex, none said the reason was because they could not access suitable services.

We asked all the sexually active female respondents what form of contraception they used and recorded up to three methods per woman. For example, a woman might use the diaphragm with spermicidal cream, which counted as two methods used together, and if she did not use the diaphragm when she was in a 'safe' part of her menstrual cycle, she was recorded as also using a 'safe period' method. We didn't ask about regularity of use or whether they occasionally failed to use their method. Table 12.1 shows the main methods of contraception used. Methods used by very few women (0.2 per cent or less) are not included in the table. These are spermicidal foam or

Table 12.1 Contraceptive methods reported by women

Method	Women (%*)
Oral contraceptive (the pill)	34
Tubal ligation or hysterectomy**	23
Male partner uses a condom	21
Male partner has had vasectomy	19
Male partner withdraws (*coitus interruptus*)	5
Safe period methods***	4
Progestogen injection (Depo-Provera)	2
Intrauterine device (IUD)	1
Progestogen implant	1
Diaphragm or cervical cap	1

* Adds up to more than 100 per cent because some women used more than one method. Non-users are not included.

** Hysterectomy is not primarily a method of contraception, but it has the effect of causing infertility.

*** Including Natural Family Planning (NFP), Billings, symptothermal and calendar rhythm methods used to guide periodic abstinence or timing of use of another method.

Source: Richters et al. 2003, *ANZJPH*, p. 213.

jelly, the female 'condom' (Femidon or Reality) and vaginal douching.

Australian women led the world in taking up oral contraceptives in the 1960s. With more than one woman in three using it, the pill is still the most popular single method, especially among women in their twenties. However, if you add vasectomy and tubal ligation together, there are more women protected from pregnancy by surgical methods than by taking the pill. Most of these women are in their forties (or even fifties), and almost none are under thirty. This reflects the popularity of permanent methods of contraception for a generation who mostly had children younger than people do nowadays, and were faced with the need for twenty-odd years of contraception after their last child was born. Tubal ligation is much more common among women in remote areas and less common in the cities. This may reflect poorer availability of contraceptive services and condoms in the bush, and possibly also the greater difficulty of obtaining a termination if any other method fails. Condom use is much lower in remote areas.

With more than one woman in three using it, the pill is still the most popular single method, especially among women in their twenties.

The condom is used by 21 per cent of women as a contraceptive method, but elsewhere in the interview 28 per cent of women said they had used a condom in the previous year. Some women apparently made the distinction between condom use for disease prevention and for contraception. Or perhaps some women used condoms occasionally but were not currently using them as a method of contraception at the time of the interview. About 8 per cent of women used withdrawal and/or safe period methods as a form of birth control.

Some women apparently made the distinction between condom use for disease prevention and for contraception.

Men and contraception

Obviously contraception is an issue for both men and women. But the responsibility for contraception is often left to the woman, especially in casual sex, and some men do not even know what method their partner uses. For this reason, the information given above is based on the methods reported by female respondents, even when the method may be used by the man (for example condom or vasectomy). It is interesting, though, to look at the differences in the replies about contraception from men and women in regular heterosexual relationships (Table 12.2). For a start, 19 per cent of men but only 11 per cent of women said no method was being used. Among those who report use of a method (ignoring the men who say they do not know what is being used), many men appear to be unaware their partner had her tubes tied or had a hysterectomy—21 per cent of women but only 14 per cent of men report this. More men (20 per cent) than women (16 per cent) say they used condoms. Perhaps some men use condoms without women noticing, but it's more likely that men are slightly overstating how diligent they are in using condoms, or the difference has arisen because men often have younger partners, those outside the scope of this survey, and condoms are used more by younger people. Few people use a diaphragm or cervical cap, but it seems that some women do so without the man being aware of it, because about sixty women but only about fifteen men said it was their method.

Table 12.2 Contraceptive methods reported by men and women in regular relationships

Method	Men (%*)	Women (%*)
Oral contraceptive (the pill)	27	30
Tubal ligation or hysterectomy**	14	21
Male partner uses a condom	20	16
Male partner has had vasectomy	18	19
Male partner withdraws (coitus interruptus)	2	3
Safe period methods***	3	3
Progestogen injection (Depo-Provera)	1	1
Intrauterine device (IUD)	1	1
Progestogen implant	<1	1
Diaphragm or cervical cap	<1	1

* Some people used more than one method.

** Hysterectomy is not primarily a method of contraception, but it has the effect of causing infertility.

*** Including Natural Family Planning (NFP), Billings, symptothermal and calendar rhythm methods used to guide periodic abstinence or timing of use of another method.

Source: Rissel et al. 2003, ANZJPH, p. 126.

How effective are these methods?

The popularity of the pill, especially among younger women who are likely to be most fertile, reflects its high effectiveness. Of a hundred women who start using the pill, only three will get pregnant in the first year of use. (This is a 'typical' rather than an ideal failure rate; it includes women who may have used the method less than perfectly, for example by missing the occasional pill and not using an alternative method.)

The next most common contraceptive method among women under forty is the condom (worn by the partner, of course). Relying on condoms alone means a 12 per cent chance of failure in a year. This is a difficult decision for young women to make: do they choose the condom, which largely protects them against sexually transmitted infections, but has a lower level of effectiveness? Or do they choose the pill, which is more effective but offers no protection against infection? Ideally, of course, the best choice is to take the pill but use condoms as well unless it's an exclusive relationship and the partner has been tested and found to be free of any infections (see Chapter 16, 'Sexually transmitted infections and safe sex'). But it can be hard to resist the temptation not to bother with a condom if you know you're not risking pregnancy, and it can also be hard for a woman to talk a man into using a condom if he knows she's on the pill.

Other mechanical and behavioural methods have higher failure rates—the diaphragm, withdrawal and safe period methods fail about 18 to 20 per cent of women using them for a year. That sounds bad, but it's still much better than using nothing—over 80 per cent of women having regular sex but using nothing get pregnant within a year. Surgical sterilisation, implants and IUDs are even more effective than the pill.

Considering the contraceptive methods used by Australian women and their expected failure rates, we would expect about 5 per cent of women to have an unplanned pregnancy each year. This would mean that over ten years of using contraception—say from age eighteen to twenty-eight—an average woman would have about a 50 per cent chance of falling pregnant. Yet far fewer women than this have had an abortion (see Chapter 11, 'Getting pregnant'). This suggests that women are choosing the most effective methods when it is most important to them not to fall pregnant, and that many unplanned pregnancies become wanted babies.

Why do some women not use contraception?

More than two thirds of women (71 per cent) use some form of contraception. We asked those who were not what the reason was and their answers are summarised in Table 12.3. The most common reason is that they are not having intercourse. Other reasons given for not using some form of contraception are being past menopause, being pregnant, trying for a baby, being infertile and/or having an infertile partner.

That leaves 13 per cent of the non-users who appeared to be at risk of unplanned pregnancy—they were having intercourse, but they weren't infertile or deliberately trying to get pregnant. These women 'at risk' gave a variety of reasons why they weren't using birth control. The most common reason was that they had side-effects or medical reasons why they could not use a method. Of course this is not really a reason for using no contraception at all, only a reason for avoiding a particular method. It suggests that doctors should always give women information about alternative methods, as a woman may give up and not come back if she has problems with a single recommended method such as the pill.

Some women said they just didn't worry about contraception—they didn't care, or just forgot, or had never got pregnant.

The next most common reason was to say, 'I leave it up to chance when to have babies', or something similar. You could regard these women as 'trying' to get pregnant without admitting it to themselves. Some of them may have been too old to have much chance of getting pregnant, even though they were not yet past menopause. Or perhaps some of them had religious reasons for leaving it to chance (or God). No one explicitly said they had religious reasons for not using contraception.

Some women said they just didn't worry about contraception—they didn't care, or just forgot, or never got pregnant. After taking a few risks and not getting pregnant, some women decide that the risk of getting pregnant on any one occasion is lower than they thought. Women

Table 12.3 Women's main reason for not using contraception

Reason given	Women (%)
Not having intercourse	42
Past menopause	22
Pregnant now	9
Want a baby	8
Respondent is infertile	5
Partner is infertile	1
Both partners infertile	1
Other	13

Source: Richters et al. 2003, *ANZJPH*, p. 212.

may even privately suspect that they are subfertile, so further risk-taking becomes a way of trying to find out. A further group of the apparently at-risk non-users said they were currently breastfeeding, though this alone may not be sufficient to cover them, especially if the baby is eating food as well and not being breastfed frequently. Some women said they thought contraception was unnatural or unhealthy. Again, they might have meant the pill or IUD when they said this, so it's not entirely clear why they did not use any method at all. It's possible too that some of these women had religious reasons for not using contraception but didn't express it that way. Very few women said the reason they didn't use contraception was because they didn't know what to do.

Given that so many Australian women use contraception, and appear to have good knowledge and access to services, most unplanned pregnancies are likely to be the result of method failure or inconsistent use, or perhaps unexpected sex.

Young people

Women under twenty were the most likely not to have a current contraceptive method even though they appeared to be at risk—10 per cent of teenagers but only 3 per cent to 6 per cent of women over twenty had no current method. However, young people were also the most likely to have intercourse only occasionally, so it's not clear from our data just how much of a risk they are taking. Pregnancy rates among teenagers have been falling since the 1970s. What is strikingly clear is that young people now take much more care the first time they have sex than their parents did. When we asked about what protection they used the first time they had intercourse, older people were much more likely than younger people to say 'nothing'. Among those who had intercourse for the first time in the late 1950s, only around 30 per cent said they used a condom or some other form of contraception. But among those who had intercourse for the first time in the late 1990s, 90 per cent used contraception (see Chapter 1, 'First times'). This would more than make up for the fact that teenagers now have first intercourse on average a year or two younger than people did in the 1950s—as long as they continue to use contraception on subsequent occasions.

Melissa, 49, believes she's used just about all the different types of contraception during the course of her sexual life. When she lost her virginity at 18 she hadn't thought about what to use. Fortunately her boyfriend pulled out—and came all over the skirt that was bunched up around her waist. After talking to friends she insisted the next boyfriend use a condom. But she couldn't understand his reluctance to use them—surely a moment of embarrassment in the chemist's shop was better than dealing with a pregnancy?

When she had her first long-term relationship in her early twenties, she went on the pill, which suited her once she found the right brand—on the first one she just didn't feel right; she never felt randy in the same way, though she had no idea how to explain this to a doctor. She used the pill off and on for the next ten years, sometimes stopping if she wasn't seeing anyone regularly, and using condoms if she had a one-night stand. Once she'd had to use the 'morning-after pill' when a condom had broken. It made her feel sick, but it was worth it: she certainly didn't want to have a baby with that guy, and wasn't even sure why she'd been attracted to him in the first place.

Then she'd met Dominic, now her husband. After they had their kids she didn't want to go back on the pill so she tried the IUD. She was always vaguely worried about having something inside her, and Dominic said he could feel the string against the tip of his penis. Eventually Dominic agreed to have a vasectomy. She felt bad when she saw him hobbling out of the day surgery clinic, but she was glad not to have her tubes tied, as that would have been a much more serious operation. Not having to think about contraception any more was a relief for them both.

Emergency contraception

Almost one in five women (19 per cent of those who have ever had intercourse) have used emergency contraception, sometimes called the morning-after pill. Half of these women have used it once only, some have used it twice and some have used it three or more times—the highest number of times reported was twelve. It sounds crazy to use emergency contraception repeatedly rather than use a regular method of contraception, but for women who have intercourse very rarely, it is not illogical compared with taking the pill day after day in months when they're not having sex. The morning-after pill can also be necessary when a condom breaks or intercourse happens unexpectedly—or against a woman's will. It is usually recommended to be taken within three days of intercourse.

Women over forty were less likely ever to have used emergency contraception, reflecting the fact that the method was not well known or easily available when those women were in their twenties. Women in remote areas, women from non-English-speaking backgrounds and those with less education were less likely to use emergency contraception. Emergency contraception is likely to be used more since the change of regulations in 2004 that made it available from a pharmacist without a doctor's prescription. It is hoped that this will reduce the need for pregnancy terminations.

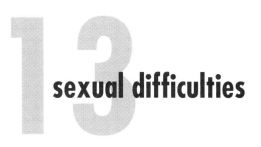

sexual difficulties

Sex may be enjoyable, but it's not perfect all the time. If you include simply not feeling like it as a difficulty, the majority of Australians have had a sexual difficulty that lasted a month or more in the year before the interview (see Table 13.1).

Table 13.1 Sexual difficulties for at least one month in the past year

Sexual difficulties	Men (%)	Women (%)
Lacked interest in having sex[1]	25	55
Came to orgasm too quickly[2]	24	12
Worried during sex about whether body looked unattractive[3]	14	36
Unable to come to orgasm[2]	6	29
Felt anxious about ability to perform sexually[3]	16	17
Did not find sex pleasurable[3]	6	27
Physical pain during intercourse[4]	2	20
Trouble with vaginal dryness[5]	–	24
Trouble keeping erection[6]	10	–
Used treatment to aid erections[6]	2	–

1 Asked of everyone
2 Asked of everyone who had any form of sex with a partner or masturbated alone
3 Asked of everyone who had any form of sex with a partner
4 Asked of everyone who had intercourse
5 Asked only of women
6 Asked only of men

Source: Richters et al. 2003, *ANZJPH*, p. 166.

Lack of interest in sex

A quarter of the men and more than half the women in the survey said they lacked interest in having sex for at least a month in the past year. Of course, we don't know whether people actually see this as a problem. If you have no partner, or your partner is ill or uninterested, you may be quite relieved that you're not constantly longing for sex you can't have. Noteworthy differences between men and women emerge when you look at the ages of people who report this difficulty (Figure 13.1). Among men, lacking interest in sex is lowest among those in their twenties and higher among men in their forties and fifties. You could speculate that this pattern largely reflects biology—men are most interested (or least likely to be uninterested) in their twenties and thirties, the peak reproductive years, when their male hormone levels are highest. However, men in their teens are more likely to say they lack interest than men in their twenties. The higher rate of lack of interest among men under twenty may be related to the sense of performance pressure experienced by many young men. This is confirmed by the age pattern for feeling anxious about sexual performance (see below).

Unlike men, women do not seem to be most interested during their peak reproductive years.

Among women, the youngest group are the *least* likely to say they lack interest. If you seek a biological explanation for this, it may lie in the fact that girls reach sexual maturity younger than boys. However, at all ages there are more women who lack interest than men. And unlike men, women do not seem to be most interested during their peak reproductive years. If the pattern were largely biological you would expect lack of interest among women to be at its lowest in their twenties, with a sharp rise in their fifties. This is not what Figure 13.1 shows us. Women report high rates of lack of interest at all ages over twenty.

For some people, a temporary lack of interest (or any other sexual difficulty) may be the result of ill health. People who say their health is excellent are least likely to have sexual difficulties in general, and those with poor health are most likely to do so. Lack of interest may also be related to exhaustion due to overwork. Since the 1990s, people have been working longer hours, and Australian research into housework has shown that even when women work full time, male partners still do only a small share of the household chores and child care.

A temporary lack of interest (or any other sexual difficulty) may be the result of ill health.

Reaching orgasm too quickly

The next most common problem for men is coming to orgasm too quickly. We don't know whether the men who complain of this actually come faster than men who do not. It may be just that they wish they could last longer. Certainly we can't tell from the survey whether men suffer from what a sex therapist would call 'premature' or 'rapid' ejaculation. Young men under twenty were (implausibly) the least likely to say they came too fast, but after that it does not change much from the twenties to the fifties.

Perhaps teenage men do not worry about coming quickly because they have not yet learnt that women may expect them to last longer, or because they recover quickly so it is not a problem. After all, coming quickly is not a physiological ailment, it is quite natural.

> **Perhaps teenage men do not worry about coming quickly because they have not yet learnt that women may expect them to last longer.**

It is just a social expectation in western culture that intercourse should be prolonged, as many people see intercourse as the central sexual act in an encounter (see Chapter 2, 'What people do'). Reaching orgasm quickly is not purely a male concern: 12 per cent of women said they came too quickly, though it was less common among the under-twenties and over-fifties.

Figure 13.1 Lack of interest in sex for at least one month in the past year

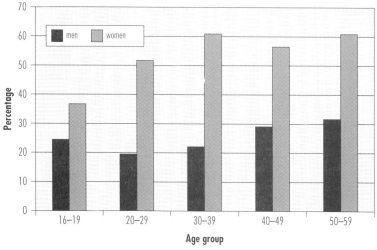

Source: Richters et al. 2003, ANZJPH, p. 167.

Worrying during sex

The second most common problem for women was worrying during sex about whether their body looked unattractive—twice as many women as men said they worried about this. This is different from worrying in general whether you will be attractive enough to get a partner. Rather it is an indicator of being self-conscious while having sex or doing what the sex therapists call 'spectatoring'—watching yourself have sex rather than enjoying yourself wholeheartedly. People worry about this less as they get older and settle down with one partner and become more comfortable with their bodies. Paradoxically, it is the young, despite being more likely to have conventionally 'attractive' bodies, who worry during sex about how they look.

Not being able to reach orgasm

For women it is common not to be able to reach orgasm—29 per cent of women but only 6 per cent of men have this difficulty. After women turn fifty, they are much more likely to report this (Figure 13.2). The increase at age fifty suggests that hormone levels may play a role. From their teens to their forties, however, women have this problem somewhat less as they get older, suggesting that at least some women learn how to achieve orgasm as they get older—or their partners learn what to do. The survey findings in Chapter 2 ('What people do') about what people did the last time they had sex point to a reason for the discrepancy between men's

People do seek to make a good impression when they have sex, especially early in a relationship.

and women's experience of orgasm. Overwhelmingly, vaginal intercourse is the main thing couples do in bed. This is a great way for most men to have an orgasm. Yet for many women, it is easier to reach orgasm through sexual practices that involve direct clitoral stimulation such as manual or oral sex. And even women who can easily reach orgasm from intercourse may be more likely to do so if they have been highly aroused by other activities.

Being anxious about performance

People tend to see sex as 'natural' or having 'flow'. Yet people do seek to make a good impression when they have sex, especially early in a relationship. This can lead to anxiety about performance. One of the few areas where women do not have more difficulty than men is in performance anxiety. Possibly this reflects social attitudes that all a woman has to do to be good is bed is to be responsive—to lie back and enjoy it.

Anxiety about sexual performance may mean different things to different people. Narrowly, 'performance' for men can mean the ability to get and keep an erection and perform intercourse. More broadly it can mean the ability to exercise sexual skill or technique for one's partner's pleasure and one's own. Despite their ease in getting and maintaining an erection compared to men over forty, young men under twenty were the most likely to report feeling anxious about performance (Figure 13.3). Confident sexual performance, it seems, is more a matter of learning and experience than of body function. No clear age patterns were apparent in women's anxiety about performance. Women's performance anxiety levels were the same as men's overall, but men seem to become less anxious as they get older and more experienced from the teens to the thirties, with anxiety levels only rising again from the forties when some start to lose interest or start having erection problems.

Figure 13.2 Not being able to reach orgasm for at least one month in the past year

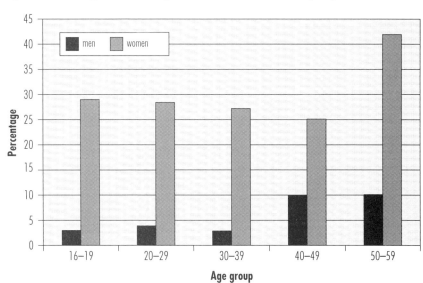

Source: Richters et al. 2003, *ANZJPH*, p. 167.

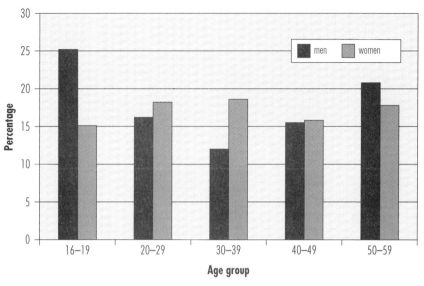

Figure 13.3 Anxiety about ability to perform sexually for at least a month in the past year

Source: Richters et al. 2003, *ANZJPH*, p. 167.

Lack of pleasure and other problems

More than a quarter of women said they did not find sex pleasurable. Only 6 per cent of men said this. Again this suggests that many women are having sex that they don't really like or want. Women are least likely to say this when they were under twenty. Men under twenty are very unlikely not to find sex pleasurable. Although men in general find sex more pleasurable than women, men aged over forty are much more likely than younger men to say they do not find sex pleasurable.

Together with not feeling like it and not enjoying it, women are also more likely to report physical problems with sex—20 per cent have physical pain during intercourse and 24 per cent have trouble with vaginal dryness. This is much higher than the 10 per cent of men who have trouble with keeping an erection. Of course, when a woman says she has pain during

> **It may be that her partner is rough or inept, or has intercourse with her when she is not aroused.**

intercourse we do not know whether there is anything physically wrong with her. It may be that her partner is rough or inept, or has intercourse with her when she is not aroused.

Although 10 per cent of men said they had trouble keeping an erection when they wanted to (for at least one month in the past year), less than 2 per cent had ever used any treatment, such as Viagra (sildenafil), and most of these were in the over-fifty age group. This survey was done before the release of the other new drugs such as Cialis (tadalafil) and Levitra (vardenafil), which work in a similar way to Viagra.

Figure 13.4 Physical pain during intercourse for at least one month in the past year

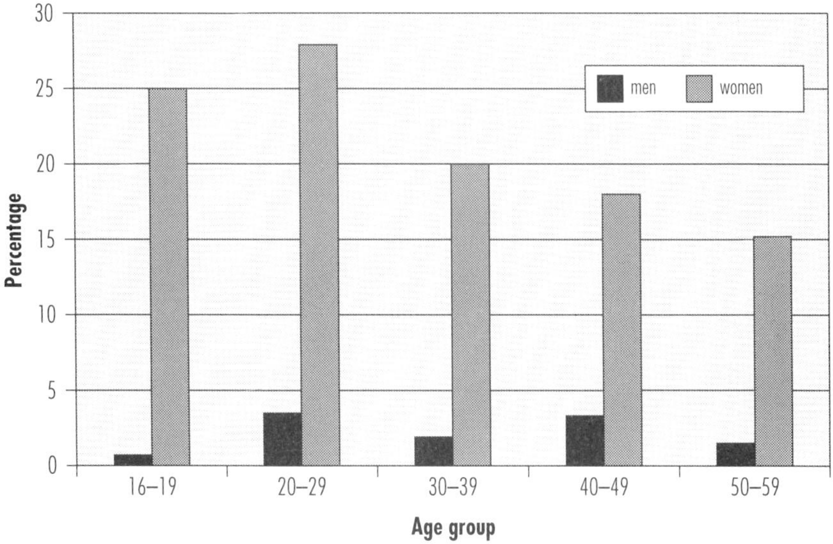

Source: Richters et al. 2003, *ANZJPH*, p. 167.

Telling an interviewer that you have one of these difficulties is not the same thing as going to the doctor with a problem or having a sex therapist make a clinical diagnosis. For example, although 24 per cent of women reported 'trouble with vaginal dryness', we do not know whether this indicates any physiological problem with vaginal lubrication, or whether it perhaps reflects a lack of desire for sex with the current partner, or lack of opportunity to become aroused before intercourse. Hormonal problems with lubrication might explain some of the trouble with dryness experienced by women past menopause and by the comparatively few women who have recently given birth.

Hormones don't, though, explain such high rates of vaginal dryness and pain during intercourse among women in their twenties and thirties. Older women were less likely to report pain during intercourse (Figure 13.4). This may be because women who find sex painful avoid it as they get older. More optimistically, it may be because couples get better at sex the longer they are together. It is still alarming that one woman in five has endured sex that she found painful for at least a month in the past year.

Joanne was 22 and had been married for three years. She loved her husband but had come to hate the sex. True, it wasn't what she married him for, but she had hoped it would improve. He was a good man, wonderful with their two-year-old son, and he had a good job—he just wasn't good in bed. She cooperated whenever he wanted sex, which didn't usually require much effort. Most of the time he'd reach over to fondle her breasts, then slide his hand down to 'warm her up' as he used to say, then roll on top of her and stick his dick into her. It was generally over pretty quickly, which was good because it often hurt. She was usually still dry when he entered her. As for having an orgasm, he didn't seem to notice that she was a long way from anything like that.

Joanne hadn't said anything to him because she didn't know what to say. All her friends seemed to have good sex lives. She just thought it would get better, like her mum had told her before they were married. The baby coming along so quickly hadn't helped things, and nor had the shift work they asked her to do at the newspaper because it would help with the child-care arrangements. Mostly she was just too tired to feel like sex, so what was the point of bothering about it?

Is it more fun for men than women?

Apart from lack of interest, men's most common problems concern timing of ejaculation and performance anxiety in general, and women's mostly concern difficulties with arousal and reaching orgasm. It is hard to avoid the conclusion that sex as it is currently practised in Australia is often more fun for men than for women.

After the striking success of Viagra—estimates suggest that since its introduction in 1998 around 130 million Viagra prescriptions have been filled, prescribed by around 600 000 doctors and used by around 16 million men—pharmaceutical companies and some sex therapists have been keen to label women's sexual problem as diseases or dysfunctions and find a drug to treat them. This is controversial because many women feel

it ignores the social and relationship reasons for women's sexual problems. Some women would no doubt love to take a pill that made them feel randier, but others feel they would enjoy sex far more if they got a chance to have the kind of sex they want. They don't want to get mended like broken sex dolls just so that they can co-operate with the kind of sex that men like best, with the emphasis on intercourse rather than sensuality and clitoral stimulation.

14 sexual assault

S adly, not all sexual activity is wanted by both the participants. While many adults might remember something they
did sexually with a bit of regret the next morning, it is very
different when someone is forced to do something sexually that
they do not want to do.

There are many definitions of sexual assault, and many
different ways of finding out how often it happens. At one
extreme there are legal definitions, such as convictions for rape
or sexual assault. However, such figures are likely to greatly
underestimate the number of assaults that actually occur. Staff
who work in sexual assault centres know that many people who
are assaulted never tell the police. Even among those who do,
not all are willing to go through the process of identifying the
perpetrator and recounting the whole ghastly experience in
court. And a conviction is not guaranteed—there may be too
little evidence, apart from what the victim says, to get the
assailant convicted.

Survey results are very useful for finding out how many
people have been sexually assaulted even if they have never
reported it. After much discussion, we chose to ask the question
'Have you ever been forced or frightened by a male or female
into doing something sexually that you did not want to do?'
We wanted wording that would not include mild sexual
harassment, or mild coercion or social pressure leading to
unenthusiastic or regretted sex. But we did want to include sex
that respondents definitely did not want and were forced into,
even if they did not think of it as rape or sexual assault in a legal
sense. And we wanted to include things that happened to both
men and women. We used the words 'male or female' rather
than 'man or woman' so as to include things done to boys or
girls by other children or teenagers.

Sobering statistics

One in five (21 per cent) Australian women have been forced or frightened into doing something sexually that they did not want to do. This experience is consistent across women of most ages and backgrounds, although older women are less likely to have had this happen to them, as are women from non-English-speaking backgrounds. Women who identify as bisexual or lesbian are much more likely to have been coerced sexually than other women. Having been sexually forced by a male in the past may well influence a woman's preference for female partners later on.

Men can also be forced or frightened into unwanted sexual activity. Overall, 5 per cent of men in the survey had been forced or frightened into doing something sexually that they did not want. Men who now identify as bisexual or gay are many times more likely to have been coerced sexually than other men. We do not know whether this is because gay and bisexual men run the risk of violence or coercion when they seek sex with other men, especially strangers, or because boys who have been sexually assaulted are more likely to grow up gay.

Because it would be difficult to help or follow up if anyone became distressed during the anonymous telephone interview, we did not ask for more details about the occasion of sexual coercion—who did it, how old they were, the circumstances, what exactly happened and so on. However, we know from other research that most people who are forced into sexual acts are forced by men. Sexual coercion of men or boys by women or girls does happen, but it is rare. It can be especially difficult for a boy to report a sexual assault, or indeed even to see the event as an assault. The macho response to the *idea* that they would have to be forced to have sex makes some men laugh. It is not so funny if you remember that the assailants are mostly men, and the victims of coercion are often boys, or men in dependent situations such as prison inmates or residents of institutions. We also know that most people are assaulted by someone they know (a family member or an acquaintance) rather than a stranger.

It can be especially difficult for a boy to report a sexual assault, or indeed even to see the event as an assault.

In the survey about half the victims of sexual coercion were sixteen or younger the first time it happened (see Table 14.1). It appears that children and people first becoming sexually active are those most vulnerable to being forced to have sex.

We did not ask the survey respondents whether they themselves had ever forced anyone to do something sexually. It's possible that some people might be prepared to admit they had done so—for example men who think it's okay to force someone in certain circumstances, say when they feel a woman has 'led them on'. However, we thought it more likely that by asking the question we would simply offend people without gaining accurate statistics on perpetrators.

Women are more likely than men to have been repeatedly forced into sex. For example, among men who had been forced or frightened into sex, 51 per cent remembered one instance of sexual forcing, and 4 per cent said that it happened too many times to count or that they could not remember how many times it happened. Sexual forcing occurred only once for 38 per cent of female victims, but 18 per cent said that it had been too frequent to count.

Remarkably, only a third of victims of sexual assault (both men and women) had talked to anyone about their experience. Some people talked about their experience to more than one person. Most commonly, people who had been sexually assaulted talked to their friends, their parents or a counsellor or psychologist. Only 4 per cent of female victims spoke to a rape crisis centre.

Table 14.1 Age when (first) forced or frightened into unwanted sexual activity*

Age when (first) coerced	Men (%)	Women (%)
<9 years	18	16
9–12 years	15	12
13–16 years	25	22
17–20 years	26	32
21–24 years	6	10
25+ years	10	9

* Among people who had ever been forced, 5% of all men and 21% of all women

Source: De Visser et al. 2003, *ANZJPH*, p. 200.

> **Remarkably, only a third of victims of sexual assault (both men and women) had talked to anyone about their experience.**

The after effects

The consequences of being a victim of sexual coercion can be devastating. Women who have experienced forced sex are more likely than other women to be anxious and unhappy, to smoke or have smoked in the past, to have injected drugs and to have had a sexually transmitted infection at some time (suggesting their sex life before or afterwards was more risky than average). Not surprisingly, the experience is also linked to less enjoyment of sex later on. Women who have been victims of sexual forcing are more likely to lack interest in sex, more likely not to find sex pleasurable, and more likely to feel anxious about their ability to perform sexually.

Men who have experienced forced sex are also more likely than other men to be anxious or unhappy, to be or have been a smoker, to have injected drugs and to have had a sexual infection at some time. Male victims of sexual forcing are, like women, more likely to lack interest in having sex, not to find sex pleasurable, and to feel anxious about their ability to perform sexually.

Angela, a twenty-year-old student and part-time IT worker, liked to go out and she had plenty of friends. She'd had a couple of semi-serious boyfriends and was not a virgin, but wasn't particularly looking for a relationship. At an office party she met Mark from the accounts department, who was talkative and pleasant and seemed attracted to her. Later that evening, Mark offered to give her a lift home.

When they arrived at her building he asked to use the toilet. She allowed him to come up to her flat, but after they came inside he locked the door and then started to take off her clothes. She protested, saying that wasn't what she had in mind, but he took no notice. He pulled off his pants and she tried to scream but then he hit her. She decided the best way not to get injured further was to let him do it, so she didn't stop him forcing himself into her. She was crying on the floor when he left. She never told anyone what happened.

paying for sex

In some cultures it used to be fairly common for an uncle or friend of the father to help 'initiate' a young man by taking him to a prostitute. The theory was that the experienced (and usually a little older) woman would teach the young man a thing or two and he would have a good start to his sex life. In practice the experience might have been a little emotionally empty but probably quite satisfying. Of course in those days young virginal women were definitely off limits, as marriage, or at least engagement, was required before a woman could be sexually active.

Today the term 'sex worker' is used instead of the somewhat demeaning or degrading term 'prostitute'. The personal services offered by sex workers have been available for millennia, and in many countries are either legal or decriminalised (do not attract serious criminal penalties). Professional sex workers treat their work very much like a regular job, and seek the same rights and benefits that other employees have.

Younger men rarely pay for sex, partly because non-commercial premarital sex is more readily available for young men than it used to be.

Men over thirty years are more likely than younger men to have ever paid for sex. Younger men rarely pay for sex, partly because non-commercial premarital sex is more readily available for young men than it used to be. The men who are more likely to have paid money for sex do not have a regular sexual partner. Interestingly, it is bisexual men who are most likely to have paid for sex, usually with a woman.

The average age at which a man first pays for sex is now about 22. It is typically a bit of an adventure—to try something new or with someone new without any strings attached. Half of the men who have paid money for sex have done so with three or fewer women. There are some men who have paid for sex with hundreds of women, but this is obviously not afford-able for everyone or particularly enjoyable for many.

Men who pay for sex are more likely than other men to take risks with their health. They tend to drink alcohol more heavily, and may have injected illicit drugs. They may be anxious or unhappy, and may have been diagnosed with a sexually trans-mitted infection at some time in their life. They are sexually adventurous, in the sense of being willing to try new things, and are likely to have had their first experience of intercourse before they were sixteen and to have tried anal intercourse with a woman.

Nationally, one in six men (16 per cent) have paid for some type of sex at least once in their lifetime. This varies quite a lot from state to state, which has something to do with the legisla-tion in each state. One in four men (27 per cent) who live in the Northern Territory have paid for sex, as have 20 per cent in Western Australia and 18 per cent in New South Wales. Men in South Australia (7 per cent) and the Australian Capital Terri-tory (11 per cent) are much less likely to have done so.

In the twelve months before the survey 2 per cent of men paid for sex. Men in their twenties are more likely to have paid for sex recently than men of other ages. Men without a regular sexual partner or who identify as bisexual or gay are also more likely to have paid for sex recently.

Less than 1 per cent of women have ever paid for sex. This is too few for us to glean any details from the survey. It appears from other research that women are rarely the purchasers of sexual services in Australia. Ads in newspapers and magazines offer paid sex to men who seek female or male or some-times transsexual partners (there is a market for services for men who like 'chicks with dicks'), but not to women. A few brothels offer male escort services to women, but this is a tiny part of the sex industry in Australia. The manager of one service told us that apart from the very occasional middle-aged European woman, the only female clients for male sex workers were themselves sex workers. After a hard but lucrative week, a sex worker can turn the tables and buy the kind of sex *she* wants for a change.

Most of the sex that men pay for is 'vanilla' sex—just vaginal intercourse, hand jobs and blow jobs.

What sort of sex do men pay for?

Most men who pay for sex choose a woman, but 3 per cent of men pay for sex with another man. The last time men paid for sex with a woman, they had vaginal intercourse (see Table 15.1). They may also have had their penis stimulated by hand and may have received oral sex. The price paid determines the services received. The majority of men touched the woman's breasts or genitals and one in four men gave oral sex (cunnilingus) to the sex worker. Anal sex was part of the encounter for 2 per cent of the men, and less than 1 per cent paid for bondage and discipline, sado-masochism or dominance and sub-mission.

Despite the impression you might get from reading the sex industry ads in sex newspapers and maga-zines, most of the sex that men pay for is 'vanilla' sex—just vaginal inter-course, hand jobs (manual stimulation) and blow jobs (oral sex).

Table 15.1 Sexual practices at men's most recent paid encounter with a woman

Sexual practice	Men (%)	Condom used (%)
Vaginal intercourse	95	98
Anal intercourse	2	100
Oral sex — fellatio	66	–
Oral sex — cunnilingus	27	–
Manual stimulation of penis by worker	90	–
Manual stimulation of woman's genitals by client	63	–
B&D, S&M or DS*	1	–

* Bondage and discipline, sado-masochism or dominance–submission

Source: Rissel et al. 2003, ANZJPH, p. 195.

How much does sex cost?

There is wide variation in what men pay for sex. It ranges from about $20 to $400. Lots of things influence the price. Customers pay most for the more unusual requests, such as bondage or dressing up or anal sex—often this has to be arranged ahead of time unless the sex worker offers this particular service regularly or as a speciality. Most brothels offer 'full service', which is a massage, oral sex and intercourse. The average price is about $120. Some massage parlours offer only massages, which are erotic and involve the worker sliding their naked body over the client and then manually stim-ulating the client to orgasm. Oral sex can also be offered by itself. The degree of comfort or luxury

Most brothels offer 'full service', which is a massage, oral sex and intercourse.

offered by the setting increases the cost, as does a longer amount of time with the worker, and sometimes how attractive or desirable the worker is.

Is paying for sex safe?

Unlike in some other countries, condoms are consistently used by most male and female sex workers in Australia, though some settings are safer than others. Among women sex workers, those working on the street or alone in private premises are less likely always to insist on condom use than those in brothels or private parlours with more than one worker. Private workers may have regular customers whom they feel they 'know' and with whom they see less need for condom protection. However, clients who request sex without condoms, or offer to pay extra for it, are acting very foolishly, especially where the other customers are likely to have sex with men, or come from countries with higher rates of HIV than Australia (such as parts of South-East Asia).

Sex with a sex worker is likely to be safer on average than sex with 'amateurs' who have multiple partners.

Sex with a sex worker is likely to be safer on average than sex with 'amateurs' who have multiple partners, as many people are not consistent in their use of condoms with casual partners (see Chapter 16, 'Sexually transmitted infections and safe sex'). Sex workers, because of their experience, are skilled users of condoms and are much less likely to have condoms break or slip off than other people.

John has been to a few sex workers in his life. He's 38, a finance analyst, and found his first experience with a street worker at 22 pretty exciting. It cost $40 in those days and was over quite quickly, but seemed something of a treat compared to masturbating.

He's tried a couple of brothels and the girls seemed cleaner and the standard of treatment was generally better. The service was usually the same—quick shower, lie on the bed for a brief massage, roll over for some oral sex (what a blast when she puts the condom on with her mouth!) and then the sex in a couple of different positions before the big orgasm. It often doesn't take very long, and paying $120 seems a lot for that.

These days he likes just the full-body massage, which goes for half an hour and includes a good and usually erotic massage with lots of body oil before the 'happy ending'. Not having intercourse makes him feel less guilty about having sex outside his marriage.

sexually transmitted infections and safe sex

While sex can be fun, and is usually necessary for having a baby, it does pose risks. In this chapter we look at how much people know about STIs (sexually transmitted infections), what STIs they have had, HIV (the AIDS virus), and whether and when people use condoms.

Knowledge of sexually transmitted infections

In this age of supposed openness about sex it is surprising that knowledge about STIs is not very good overall. Try yourself on this quick quiz—just answer true or false.

1. People who have injected drugs are at risk for hepatitis C
   True ❐   False ❐

2. Hepatitis C can be transmitted by tattooing and body piercing
   True ❐   False ❐

3. Hepatitis C has no long-term effects on your health
   True ❐   False ❐

4. Cold sores and genital herpes can be caused by the same virus
   True ❐   False ❐

5. Once a person has caught genital herpes, they will always have the virus
   True ❐   False ❐

6. Hepatitis B can be transmitted sexually
   True ❐   False ❐

7. Gonorrhoea can be transmitted through oral sex
   True ❐   False ❐

8. Chlamydia can lead to infertility in women
True ☐   False ☐

9. Genital warts can only be spread by intercourse
True ☐   False ☐

10. Chlamydia affects only women
True ☐   False ☐

How did you go? See Table 16.1 for the answers.

The average score is about six correct out of 10. Younger people, especially men, have the worst scores, followed by people from non-English-speaking backgrounds. Overall, women have better knowledge about sexual health than men, and this is consistent with women having better health knowledge generally. People who score highest are those who have had an STI, gay men and lesbians, and people with education beyond high-school level.

Most people got the questions about hepatitis C right, perhaps because it's easy to guess that people who have injected drugs are at risk of something, even if you've never heard of it before. The hepatitis C virus is easier to catch from

Table 16.1 Knowledge about STIs and hepatitis

		Correct response	Men (%)	Women (%)
1	People who have injected drugs are at risk for hepatitis C	True	87	85
2	Hepatitis C can be transmitted by tattooing and body piercing	True	73	73
3	Hepatitis C has no long-term effects on your health	False	69	75
4	Cold sores and genital herpes can be caused by the same virus	True	65	71
5	Once a person has caught genital herpes, they will always have the virus	True	61	75
6	Hepatitis B can be transmitted sexually	True	59	60
7	Gonorrhoea can be transmitted through oral sex	True	54	54
8	Chlamydia can lead to infertility in women	True	34	57
9	Genital warts can only be spread by intercourse	False	40	45
10	Chlamydia affects only women	False	30	32

Source: Grulich et al. 2003a, ANZJPH, p. 231.

blood-to-blood contact than HIV. There is no vaccine against it. About 75 per cent of people who catch hepatitis C become chronically infected—i.e. their immune system does not clear the virus from the body. Up to a quarter of people with hepatitis C suffer from liver diseases such as cirrhosis or liver cancer in later life. About 250 000 Australians—more than 1 per cent of the population—are thought to be infected with hepatitis C.

Genital herpes and cold sores are caused by the same virus. There are two types of the virus, one of which has been associated mainly with cold sores and the other with genital infections. Nowadays, however, it is common for people to have either type in either location. This is probably because more people have oral sex and fewer people acquire non-sexual oral herpes in childhood. It is also possible to have both types at once. People who get cold sores should avoid kissing or oral sex when they have an outbreak. People with genital herpes should use condoms, and avoid sex during outbreaks. Antiviral drugs can reduce the risk of transmitting the virus.

Hepatitis B is caused by a different virus from hepatitis C, and it is often passed on through sex, which appears to be rare for hepatitis C. Happily, there is a vaccine against hepatitis B infection.

Gonorrhoea is caused by bacteria that usually infect the man's urethra (the tube through the penis) or the woman's vagina or cervix. But the bacteria can also infect the throat and be passed on by fellatio or cunnilingus. Gonorrhoea is cured by antibiotics.

Chlamydia, like gonorrhoea, is a bacterial infection that can cause a discharge from the penis or vagina, though people can also have it without any symptoms. Unfortunately it can travel up through a woman's cervix and infect the tubes that carry the eggs from the ovaries to the uterus. If these tubes get inflamed and gummed up the woman may become infertile. Chlamydia can be cured by a course of antibiotics. Both gonorrhoea and chlamydia can be prevented by condom use.

Genital warts are caused by viruses. There is a host of related viruses that cause ordinary lumpy warts on the body, visible genital warts and also the invisible flat wart virus infections that are sometimes picked up on Pap smears. Genital wart viruses thrive in a moist environment but do not require intercourse to pass from one person to another; any close contact will do.

To find out more about HIV and other STIs and how to have safe sex, see 'References and further reading'.

Experience of sexually transmissible infections

In the survey, 20 per cent of men and 17 per cent of women said they'd had an STI, and about 2 per cent of men and women had an STI in the twelve months before our survey. The commonest STI is really an infestation rather than an infection: pubic lice, otherwise known as crabs. The next most common STIs are genital warts, followed by chlamydia and genital herpes. Half of the people who get an STI see a GP first, and the rest go to a specialist sexual health clinic, treat themselves or consult a pharmacist.

In general, the older people are, the more likely they are ever to have had an STI, because they have had more chance to be exposed to risk. However, people over fifty are less likely than people in their forties ever to have had an STI, which suggests that the over-fifty generation have led less risky sex lives—they mostly had fewer partners than the people now in their forties. Gay men have much higher rates of STIs, and this reflects their access to anonymous sex in sex clubs, gay saunas and even public toilets as well as with men they meet through friends, the Internet or gay bars. In general, having more partners puts you at more risk. Better educated people in managerial and professional jobs were slightly more likely to have ever had an STI—though this may be partly because they recognised the names of diseases in the interview questions better than other people.

The commonest STI is really an infestation rather than an infection: pubic lice, otherwise known as crabs.

The survey results are probably an underestimate of how many Australians have had an STI (or still have it, in the case of incurable infections such as herpes and HIV). Many people have had an STI without knowing it, and others may once have known they had something but forgotten. Percentage estimates vary, but it's likely that the majority of people with herpes do not know they have it, because symptoms vary from person to person—some are very ill, some have obvious blisters, and others notice nothing wrong. Women and sometimes men with gonorrhoea or chlamydia can have no symptoms at all. Women with vaginal infections and men with inflammation of the urethra may know only that they had an infection, and not what it was called.

HIV (the AIDS virus)

Forty per cent of both men and women have had an HIV test. Not surprisingly, gay men are more than twice as likely to have been tested as straight men. For women, being lesbian or bisexual seemed to have no effect on whether they had been for an HIV test or not. Very few people in our survey were HIV-positive (that is, infected with HIV)—just over one in a thousand.

Rates of HIV infection in Australia are low compared with some nearby countries. From national surveillance we know that about 13 000 people—that's six people in every 10 000— are currently living with HIV. Over 80 per cent of these are men who have had sex with other men. Others are men and women who have caught the virus through heterosexual sex, or through injecting drugs and sharing a needle. Among heterosexuals, infection is more likely among people who come from countries with high infection rates, people who have sexual partners from high-risk countries (or who have had sex overseas), and people who inject drugs.

Because HIV rates are low here, few Australians know someone who is infected. The risk seems distant, so people tend to disregard it unless they are gay. Even in the gay community, HIV is not as visible as it was in the 1980s and early 1990s. With new treatments, many infected men remain well. To some gay men it can even seem that HIV is a manageable chronic disease, something you can live with like asthma or diabetes. In recent years there has been an

Because HIV rates are low here, few Australians know someone with the virus.

increase in the number of gay men having unprotected sex, at least sporadically, but arguments continue in HIV research about whether men are taking more risks because they are less afraid of infection or for some other reason.

Certainly for gay men, after the ravages of AIDS—many gay men lost friends in the 1980s—STIs other than HIV can seem trivial. It is hard to worry too much about a sore throat or a bit of a discharge, easily fixed with antibiotics, as long as you are still HIV negative. This attitude ignores two facts. One is that the sexual acts through which you catch gonorrhoea or chlamydia are the same ones that transmit HIV. Gay men who catch STIs are taking risks: their sexual practice is not safe enough to protect them from HIV. The other is that if you have another STI, or currently have a sore from a herpes infection, your chance of catching HIV rises.

Condom use

Despite condoms being an excellent way to reduce risks of catching or passing on an STI, there are many reasons (or excuses) men give for why they do not use them. 'They reduce sensation', 'Putting it on breaks the flow and spoils the moment', 'They break', or 'I'll pull out in time'. This last action can be reasonably effective as a contraceptive (though perhaps over-optimistic for an adolescent or anyone's first time with a new partner), but it is useless to prevent STIs.

Many sexually active people do have some idea of the risks of unsafe sex. People are more likely always to use condoms with casual partners than with regular partners, and least likely to use them for sex with regular live-in partners (see Table 16.2). But there's still lots of unsafe sex going on, and that means lots of opportunities for sexually transmitted bugs to have flourishing careers. More than half of men and two thirds of women don't always use condoms with a casual opposite-sex partner.

There's lots of unsafe sex going on, and that means lots of opportunities for sexually transmitted bugs to flourish.

Table 16.2 Always used condom in the past six months

| Partner type | Vaginal intercourse | | Anal intercourse with man |
	Men (%)	Women* (%)	Men (%)
Regular live-in partner	8	6	23
Regular non-live-in partner	29	17	38
Casual partner(s)	45	35	87

* Condom worn by partner

Source: De Visser et al. 2003, *ANZJPH*, p. 226.

Men who do not always use condoms with casual female sexual partners are likely to drink a lot and to work in a blue-collar job. For women there is no single factor related to low condom use.

Billy liked to go to the pub after work with his mates from the building site. Friday night was particularly good, because he didn't have to be at work by 7 a.m. the next day. Often the girls from the office block nearby came in and stayed on for some dancing later.

One Friday night Billy found himself getting on very well with Pam, whom he hadn't met before. They had quite a lot to drink, but not enough to dampen the erection Billy had. One thing led to another and they got a taxi back to Pam's place. Her flatmate was still out and Billy started kissing and cuddling with Pam, who was very responsive. Her obvious enjoyment at being kissed just increased when he started brushing his hand across her breasts and undoing her shirt buttons. By the time he was stroking her upper thighs and dipping his fingers into her, she was as wet as anyone he'd ever been with and he could feel her heat.

They moved into Pam's room so that her flatmate didn't walk in and find them on the couch. He let her rip the buttons off his shirt as she quickly undressed him. They lay naked on her bed and as he licked and kissed her nipples he felt himself sliding between her thighs. Pam started to say something about protection but Billy didn't want to slow down. The condoms he'd bought from the machine in the pub were in his jacket pocket, but he'd left the jacket in the living room. He could pull out before he came. He just shifted a little and pushed and then he was inside her. She groaned with pleasure and they just moved together, gradually getting faster until Pam started shuddering and it was all Billy could do to hold on before he pushed himself off her and came over her belly.

After a couple of weeks Billy felt like he was getting the flu and then a watery blister appeared on his penis. He went to the doctor, who told him after getting the test results that it was genital herpes.

Safe sex and regular relationships

The gay community is much more aware of STI risks, and rightly concerned about HIV, and this is reflected in the much higher rates of condom use among men having anal intercourse than among men having sex with women.

In the gay community, many men who live together or have long-term committed relationships know they will still be tempted to have sex with other men—after all, casual sex is readily available for gay men and is a favourite pastime for some of them. When AIDS came along, health authorities recommended that the safest thing was for all gay men always to use condoms, with their regular partners as well as when they had casual sex. The trouble with this advice is that people who are in love want to be close and have sex without worrying about infection. Many people—gay and straight—feel that a condom is an emotional barrier as well as a physical one in sex: it gets in the way of the sense that 'the two of us become one'. So gay men started making deals with their regular partners. Some couples agreed to have anal sex only with each other, though touching other men, and maybe oral sex, was permitted. Some couples agreed that even anal sex outside the relationship could be okay as long as a condom was used. If there was a slip-up, they agreed to tell each other so they could use condoms in their sex at home with each other until they had both had HIV tests and got the all-clear.

When the AIDS prevention organisations realised what was going on they ran campaigns to encourage men in regular relationships to do this properly. It's not safe to just assume that because you're in love the other person (1) is uninfected and (2) won't have sex with anyone else. One campaign in Sydney was called 'Talk—test—test—trust'. This stood for talking about what the agreement in the relationship would be, getting tested for HIV twice and sharing the results, and then trusting each other to tell if anything unsafe happened outside the relationship.

Few heterosexual couples make this sort of 'negotiated safety' agreement explicitly. Many seem unaware of the risks they take by going from one partner to another without having check-ups. Doctors say that couples in new relationships sometimes make an appointment for tests before ceasing condom use, but they often ask to be tested only for HIV and not for infections that are much more common among the general population, such as chlamydia.

> **The most common way for condoms to fail is for them not to be used.**

Condom problems

Although condoms are reasonably reliable as contraceptives and using one is the best way to avoid getting or passing on an STI, condoms are not 100 per cent perfect. No method is, except abstinence (if you can stick to it). The most common way for condoms to fail is for them not to be used. It can be hard to tactfully pick the right moment to grasp the condom packet, get it open and get the condom on. When people are drunk or nervous or emotionally overwhelmed they often don't manage it.

Even when condoms are used, they sometimes tear (break) or slip off during sex. This can be a disaster for the people who have gone to the trouble of using 'protection' only to find the method failed. In the survey, over a third (37 per cent) of men who have ever used a condom have had at least one condom breakage in their lifetime. Men in their twenties are most likely to report condom breakage (47 per cent), with older men less likely to do so. Of men who used a condom in the past year, 24 per cent had a condom break. Men over thirty are less likely to have had a condom break in the past year, partly because they use fewer condoms than younger men. The more condoms you use, the greater your chance of eventually encountering a faulty one. On the other hand, an important reason younger men have more condoms break is because they often have less experience using them.

From all the research on condoms done in the past twenty years, it is clear that practice makes perfect. Beginners tend to break condoms, and people with lots of experience, such as sex workers, hardly ever have failures. Using an old condom that has been sitting around in the car or your wallet is risky (though better than no condom at all). Vigorous or prolonged intercourse can also increase the likelihood of a condom breaking. Additional lubricant is not usually needed for vaginal intercourse, but necessary for anal intercourse. Oil-based lubricants such as baby oil or hand cream may damage the condom.

Another problem with condoms is that they can slip off during or after sex. This may be caused by a slight loss of erection or penis shrinkage after orgasm. About 18 per cent of men who have used a condom in the past year have had one slip off during intercourse or during withdrawal. It's important to hold onto the rim of the condom while pulling out after intercourse. It's also important to have the condom on before there is any genital contact, if it is to be effective in preventing STI transmission. Yet of people who used a condom the last time they had sex, 13 per cent put the condom on late.

The good news is that even though quite a few men have had a condom break on them, for most it only happens once or twice. This may be because some people stop using condoms for fear it will happen again. Nonetheless, the relatively low overall failure rate makes condoms considerably less risky than unprotected intercourse. We couldn't tell from the survey how many condoms fail, but from other studies we know that between 1 and 3 per cent of condoms break, depending on who is using them.

Jim, 23, has been going out with Tina now for over six months. They get on really well and both like to be pretty wild in the cot. Jim promised Tina a massage the next time he cooked. After dinner, when the time came, he laid her down naked on a towel on the bed. He rubbed the oil in his hands first to warm it up and then started on her back. He has strong hands and he took his time massaging her neck and shoulders, arms and back, making sure to slide his fingers up and down her sides and almost touching her breasts. He stroked her buttocks and the backs of her legs, slowly sliding his fingers along the insides of her upper thighs.

By the time he turned her over and worked his way up from her feet to her waist she was ready for him. He'd had half an erection since the moment he'd touched her and didn't need much encouragement. He reached for the condoms they'd put by the bed and using both hands tore open the packet. (Tearing them with his teeth, he'd discovered earlier, could rip the condom.) He rolled it on with his oily hands and then went into her. After half a dozen different positions and some wild pumping, he could feel his orgasm building. He pumped harder. Suddenly he thought he could feel her get even hotter and then he couldn't hold on any longer and he came.

After he rolled off her, he reached down to pull off the condom and to his horror he found that only half of it was still there around the base of his penis. The condom had broken.

17 sex in Australia

Key findings

Age at first sex

- For men, the median age at first vaginal intercourse (the age at which 50 per cent of the population has had sex) has gone down over the past forty years from eighteen to sixteen among men, and from nineteen to sixteen among women.
- Contraceptive use at first intercourse has increased significantly, from less than 30 per cent of men and women in the 1950s to over 90 per cent in 2000.

Sexual identity, experience and behaviour

- Among men, 97 per cent identify as heterosexual, 2 per cent as gay or homosexual and 1 per cent as bisexual.
- Among women, 98 per cent identify as heterosexual, 1 per cent as lesbian or homosexual and 1 per cent as bisexual.
- Some same-sex attraction or experience is reported by 9 per cent of men and 15 per cent of women.
- Men and women who identify as homosexual (gay or lesbian) or bisexual report more sexual partners than people who identify as heterosexual.

Heterosexual behaviour

- Men say they've had more sexual partners than women over their lifetime, in the past five years, and in the past year.
- Fifteen per cent of men and 9 per cent of women have had more than one sexual partner in the past year.
- At their most recent heterosexual encounter, almost everyone had vaginal intercourse. Oral sex has become more popular among younger age groups.
- Anal intercourse (among heterosexuals) was uncommon—

21 per cent of men and 15 per cent of women have ever had it, and only 1 per cent did it the last time they had sex.

- Some people never have sex—8 per cent in the survey have never had vaginal intercourse, and about 3 per cent will never have intercourse in their lifetimes. Only a minority of these people are gay or lesbian.
- Even with casual partners, only a minority (45 per cent of men, 35 per cent of women) always use condoms for intercourse.

Regular relationships

- Seventy-four per cent of men and 77 per cent of women are in a regular heterosexual relationship.
- In the four weeks before being interviewed, men and women in regular relationships had sex with their partners an average of 1.8 times per week.
- Most respondents expect themselves and their partners to not have sex with other people, although men are less likely than women to have discussed these expectations with their partner.
- Five per cent of men and 3 per cent of women in regular heterosexual relationships have had sex with someone other than their regular partners in the past twelve months.

Contraception

- Seventy-one per cent of the population use some method of contraception.
- The most common reasons for not using contraception are not having intercourse and being past menopause.
- Among women who appear to be at risk of unplanned pregnancy, the most common reasons for not using contraceptives are experience of side-effects or contraindications, leaving it to chance and forgetting or not caring. Some women are breastfeeding and some believe contraception to be unnatural or unhealthy.
- The most commonly used contraceptive methods reported by women are oral contraceptives (34 per cent of users), tubal ligation/hysterectomy (23 per cent), condoms worn by the partner (21 per cent) and vasectomy of partner (19 per cent).

Fertility

- Among women, 16 per cent have experienced difficulty in becoming pregnant.

- Seventy-six per cent have been pregnant at least once, and most of these women have had a live birth.
- Of women who have been pregnant, 33 per cent have experienced a miscarriage and 23 per cent have had a termination of pregnancy.
- Fewer women become pregnant for the first time as teenagers nowadays—23 per cent of women in their fifties and 17 per cent of women in their twenties were pregnant before age twenty.

Difficulties
- The most common sexual difficulty is lack of interest in having sex (25 per cent of men, 55 per cent of women).
- Women are more likely than men to report
  - being unable to come to orgasm (29 per cent compared with 6 per cent of men)
  - not finding sex pleasurable (27 per cent of women, 6 per cent of men)
  - physical pain during intercourse (20 per cent of women, 2 per cent of men)
  - worrying during sex about their body looking unattractive (36 per cent of women, 14 per cent of men).
- Men are more likely than women to report coming to orgasm too quickly (24 per cent compared with 12 per cent of women).
- Men (16 per cent) and women (17 per cent) are equally likely to have felt anxious about their ability to perform sexually.
- Erectile difficulties in men and lack of interest in sex are higher among those over forty.
- Anxiety about performance is highest among men under twenty.

Satisfaction
- Most people in heterosexual relationships find sex very or extremely pleasurable (90 per cent of men, 79 per cent of women) and the relationship emotionally satisfying (88 per cent of men, 79 per cent of women).
- People who find the sex in their relationship physically pleasurable are likely to be emotionally satisfied as well.
- One person in four has had no sex in the past four weeks; most people have sex less than twice a week.
- Most people (both men and women) want ideally to have sex more often than they are having it.

- A quarter of men (24 per cent) but only 8 per cent of women say they ideally want sex daily or more often.

Masturbation and other sexual pursuits
- Sixty-five per cent of men and 35 per cent of women have masturbated in the past year.
- Nearly half (48 per cent) of the men and 25 per cent of the women have masturbated in the past four weeks. Among these people, men did so 5.8 times on average and women 3.3 times.
- About a quarter of all respondents have watched an X-rated film (37 per cent of men, 16 per cent of women) in the past year.
- Seventeen per cent of men and 2 per cent of women have visited an Internet sex site in the past year.
- Twelve per cent of men and 14 per cent of women have used a sex toy in the last year.
- Seventeen per cent of men and 14 per cent of women have engaged in digital anal stimulation with a partner in the past year.
- Phone sex, role play or dressing up, bondage and discipline, and other anal practices (fisting and rimming) were engaged in by less than 5 per cent of the sample.

Sex work
- About one man in six (16 per cent) has ever paid for sex; 2 per cent have done so in the past year.
- Of men who have ever paid for sex, 97 per cent paid for sex with a woman and 3 per cent for sex with a man.
- Very few women (0.1 per cent) have ever paid for sex.
- Condom use during sex was highest at parlours, brothels and with escorts, and lowest with street sex workers.

Sexual assault
- Twenty-one per cent of women and 5 per cent of men reported experience of sexual coercion—being forced or frightened into sexual activity—and 3 per cent of men and 10 per cent of women reported sexual coercion when aged sixteen or younger.
- Few people had talked to others about their experiences of sexual coercion and fewer had talked to a professional.

Attitudes
- Most people agree that premarital sex is acceptable, that

oral sex counts as 'sex', that sex is important for a sense of wellbeing, and that extramarital sex is unacceptable. Men are more likely (37 per cent) to disapprove of sex between two men than women are to disapprove of sex between two women (25 per cent).

- People with higher levels of education tend to have more tolerant views.

Sexually transmitted infections

- Knowledge of infections such as herpes, gonorrhoea, genital warts and chlamydia is limited.
- Women have better knowledge about sexually transmitted infections than men.
- Twenty per cent of men and 17 per cent of women have ever been diagnosed with an STI, with 2 per cent of both men and women being diagnosed with an STI in the past year.
- Most people go to their usual GP for treatment. Others go to a pharmacist or a sexual health clinic.
- Forty per cent of men and women have been tested for HIV. Among gay men, 77 per cent have been tested.

How do we compare with other countries?

A natural question that often arises after looking at the results of our survey is 'How different are we from people in other countries?' This question is much harder to answer than you might think, because surveys in other countries ask slightly different questions and analyse the answers differently. However, we can make some broad generalisations.

Age at first sex

As in Australia, surveys in Europe and America have found that over the past few decades people have become sexually active at slightly earlier ages. This fall in the age at first intercourse has been greater for women than for men. (Or perhaps women have become more ready to admit to early sex.)

Use of contraception during the first time young people have sex is more common here than in the United States, where overall 34 per cent of men and 38 per cent of women reported they used some form of contraception the first time they had intercourse. Teenage pregnancy rates in Australia are also much lower than in the United States or Britain, though higher than in many European countries, so we have much room for improvement.

Homosexual and bisexual identity, attraction and behaviour

Research from other developed Western countries suggests that approximately 98 per cent of men and women describe their sexual identity as 'heterosexual', with the remaining 2 per cent split between 'bisexual', 'homosexual' and 'other/undecided' categories. At the same time, approximately 8 per cent of adults in overseas studies say that in terms of sexual attraction and/or experience they are not exclusively heterosexual (or indeed at all). The proportion of respondents with some same-sex experience ranges from 1 per cent of Portuguese men to 12 per cent of Dutch men, and from 1 per cent of Portuguese women to 9 per cent of Finnish women. In most countries, men were more likely than women to report homosexual experience. Australia differs from this pattern in that more women (9 per cent) than men (6 per cent) report having some same-sex experience. The proportion of men who report homosexual activity in the past year ranges from 1.1 per cent in France and Britain to 6.3 per cent in the Netherlands, while for women this varies from 0.3 per cent in France to 1.3 per cent in the United States.

Some of the studies allowed comparisons of sexual attraction and sexual experience. In the 1990 British survey, 90 per cent of men and 92 per cent of women said they were exclusively heterosexual in terms of attraction and experience. Looking at this the other way around, we see that 10 per cent of men and 8 per cent of women reported some homosexual attraction and/or experience. The proportion of British respondents who were exclusively homosexual in both attraction and experience was 0.3 per cent for men and 0.1 per cent for women. In the French survey, 7 per cent of men and 16 per cent of women reported homosexual attraction and/or experience, while in the Netherlands, 14 per cent of men and 6 per cent of women reported some homosexual attraction and/or experience.

These results are broadly similar to those in Australia, although the percentage of women here who report some same-sex attraction (13 per cent) is at the high end of the range. More generally, Australia seems to conform to a pattern common in northern Europe and in other English-speaking countries in which the existence of homosexuality in men and women is acknowledged and widely accepted, despite the existence of prejudice. In many of these countries discrimination against homosexuals is discouraged or even illegal. However, people are largely expected to be either straight or gay, and this is especially true for men. Same-sex activity by men who identify as heterosexual is puzzling or even alarming to many Australians. Bisexuality is not widely recognised as a valid sexual identity and is not protected by discrimination legislation.

Heterosexual relationships and partner numbers

Internationally, about half of the population have had sex with fewer than five opposite-sex partners over their lifetimes, while approximately 30 per cent of men and 10 per cent of women report 10 or more sexual partners. In the British study, over 90 per cent of respondents reported heterosexual activity in the past year—approximately three-quarters of respondents had sex with only one partner, and less than 5 per cent of men and 2 per cent of women reported five or more sexual partners. As in Australia, men were more likely to report multiple partners than women, and younger people reported more recent partners than older people.

In Australia, 5 per cent of men and 3 per cent of women in regular heterosexual relationships had sex with someone else in the previous twelve months. These rates are generally lower than those reported in European countries in the late 1980s and early 1990s (among men, 6 per cent in Britain, 8 per cent in France and the Netherlands, and 10 per cent in Belgium and Norway; among women, 2 per cent in Great Britain, 3 per cent in the Netherlands, 4 per cent in France and Belgium and 6 per cent in Norway). However, these figures are not directly comparable to the Australian results because the questions were asked in different ways.

The British survey done in 2000 appears to report high rates of 'concurrency' (i.e. sex with more than one partner in the same period)—15 per cent of men and 9 per cent of women. However, most of the difference between Britain and Australia is due to the different way in which this was measured in the British survey, which counted any overlap of partners as 'concurrency'. In other words, if a single woman had casual sex with Tony in April and Brian in June, then Tony again in September, she was counted as having concurrent partners. This was reported in the media as 'cheating'. In our study only people who had sex with someone else while they were in a regular relationship that had lasted more than a year were counted as 'playing around'—and not all of them were cheating in the sense of deceiving their partners. The British figures, however, were very similar to our rates for people with two or more partners in the previous year, so the difference is largely one of definition. It does seem that Australians are committed to the notion of sexual exclusivity when they are in a relationship, and they are more likely to stick to this commitment than Europeans.

Contraception

In the US national survey, 53 per cent of men and 47 per cent of women reported they always used some form of contraception during intercourse with their primary partner. Sixty-nine per cent of men and women used contraception at least some of the time. That study also revealed that 38 per cent of women were sterile (29 per cent had been sterilised by choice), as were 13 per cent of men (12 per cent had been sterilised by choice). Among both women and men, the prevalence of voluntary sterilisation was very low among young people and increased with age: more than 40 per cent of women aged over forty had been sterilised by choice. Although the overall rate of contraceptive use is similar to Australia, the rates of female sterilisation in the United States appear higher than here, though the vasectomy rates are lower. The difference may be due to the high cost of private health care in America and the fact that some public clinics offer free or subsidised sterilisation.

In the 1990 British national survey, among respondents who reported at least one heterosexual partner in the previous year, 79 per cent of women and 82 per cent of men reported use of a method of contraception. Some of those reporting no method may have been pregnant, seeking pregnancy, or sterile for non-contraceptive reasons. Less than 10 per cent of sexually active people were unprotected against unplanned pregnancy. The forms of contraception most commonly used in the previous year were the pill (reported by 30 per cent of men, 29 per cent of women), condoms (37 per cent of men, 26 per cent of women) and male or female sterilisation (21 per cent of men, 23 per cent of women). These figures are similar to Australia, although slightly more women here use the pill (34 per cent) and somewhat fewer report that their partner uses condoms (21 per cent). Given the similarities in our health care systems, and the fact that condoms are widely available from pharmacies and vending machines in both countries, the similar patterns are not surprising.

Fertility

The US national survey done in 1990–91 revealed that 72 per cent of women had given birth. That study also showed that

76 per cent of conceptions reported by women resulted in a live birth, with 13 per cent resulting in miscarriage, 10 per cent being aborted, and fewer than 1 per cent resulting in a stillbirth. These rates are similar to Australia, though in our survey the question was asked slightly differently—first it asked women whether they had ever been pregnant (76 per cent). Among the pregnancies (conceptions) reported in Australia there were slightly fewer live births (72 per cent) and more miscarriages (17 per cent). In America, as in Australia, younger women were more likely to report having had an abortion than older women. Among women with more education a higher proportion of pregnancies were terminated. Termination rates were not the same for all age groups—women aged under twenty and women aged over forty reported the highest proportion of pregnancies terminated. Termination rates also increased over time, from 2 per cent of conceptions in the 1950s to 18 per cent in the 1990s. It is interesting that despite the high-profile opposition to abortion from some religious groups in the United States—clinics have been bombed and doctors murdered—the same proportion of pregnancies are aborted there as in Australia.

In the British national survey in 1990, 6 per cent of men and 8 per cent of women (about the same as in our study) reported that they or their partner had sought professional help for infertility. The British study revealed that 21 per cent of women had experienced a miscarriage or stillbirth, and 12 per cent of women had had an induced abortion. Both these figures appear lower than in Australia (26 per cent and 16 per cent respectively), although the reasons for this are unclear.

Sexual difficulties

The United States national survey found that women (33 per cent) were more likely than men (16 per cent) to report lack of interest in sex, inability to come to a climax (24 per cent of women and 8 per cent of men), lack of pleasure during sex (21 per cent of women and 8 per cent of men), and pain during intercourse (14 per cent of women and 3 per cent of men). In contrast, men (29 per cent) were more likely than women (10 per cent) to report climaxing too soon and anxiety about performance (17 per cent of men and 12 per cent of women). In addition, 19 per cent of women reported difficulty lubricating, and 10 per cent of men reported inability to get or keep an erection. These results are similar to ours, except that in Australia there was no gender difference in performance anxiety.

In the Danish national survey, 30 per cent of women and 27 per cent of men reported a current sexual problem. Among women the most common problems were 'reduced desire' (11 per cent of women) and lack of orgasm (7 per cent). Among men the most frequently reported problems were difficulty achieving an erection (5 per cent) and premature ejaculation (5 per cent). A survey of Swedish adults revealed that in the year prior to the survey 23 per cent of men and 47 per cent of women reported at least one sexual difficulty. In that study 16 per cent of men and 34 per cent of women had lacked interest in sex, 12 per cent of women had problems with lubrication, 5 per cent of men had erectile difficulties, 9 per cent reported premature ejaculation, and 1 per cent of men and 6 per cent of women reported pain during intercourse. For men, problems of desire, erection, ejaculation and pain were relatively infrequent until after age fifty. Young women were less likely than older women to report lack of interest, problems with lubrication, or pain. Men and women in relationships were less likely to report lack of interest in sex, and various other sexual difficulties.

Overall, although the figures are somewhat different from country to country because the questions differ somewhat, the pattern is similar. Women are more likely to report lack of interest, pain and lack of pleasure in sex than men. Arguments will continue to rage over whether this is because there is biologically 'something wrong' with women (or something wrong with men for hurting them), or because roughly similar social arrangements and sexual conventions apply in all these Western countries.

Sex work

Surveys in Europe reveal great variety in the proportion of men who have paid for sex in their lives—from 7 per cent in Britain to 39 per cent in Spain, with the average figure around 15 per cent. The proportion of men who have paid for sex in the previous year also varies, from 1 per cent in Britain to 11 per cent in Spain, with an average of around 2 to 3 per cent. Countries have very different legal approaches to sex work, from the Netherlands where sex workers are treated like other workers, to Sweden, which has experimented with outlawing sex work entirely and arresting would-be customers. In some countries sex work is technically illegal but in fact carried out more or less openly. Where prostitution is illegal, people may be less willing to admit to survey researchers that they have paid for sex.

The results from our survey put Australia in an average position internationally.

Sexual assault

Studies of representative samples in the United States reveal that approximately 20 per cent of women and 5 per cent of men have experienced sexual coercion. These rates are almost identical to those in Australia. Rates of sexual coercion are not readily available from many countries.

Sexually transmissible infections

Studies in New Zealand, the United States, Finland, the Netherlands and Norway suggest that 10 to 20 per cent of adults have been diagnosed with an STI at some point in their lives. In the 2000 British survey, 11 per cent of men and 13 per cent of women who had had intercourse reported having ever had an STI. The Australian results are at the high end of the range.

Conclusion

The Australian Study of Health and Relationships achieved a large sample and a high response rate. It documented the sexual knowledge, attitudes and practices of the Australian population aged 16 to 59. Because the results are only a snapshot of what is happening, we cannot explain exactly why some behaviours or attitudes are more common than others.

Young Australians start having sex earlier than their parents did, but they are more likely to use contraception than their parents when they first had intercourse. Many Australians are in regular relationships, and they have sex, on average, a couple of times a week. Most of these people say they enjoy the sex they have and that they are emotionally satisfied in their relationships. However, we also found that almost half of the men and almost three-quarters of the women in the survey said they had experienced some form of sexual difficulty for at a least a month in the previous year. These difficulties may not in themselves be problems for people, but they are certainly a common experience. Women's experience of sex was generally less positive than men's.

The high levels of sexual assault or coercion are of significant concern. Few of the people who had been forced into sex had talked about their experience to others, and even fewer had talked to a counsellor.

This study was the first large-scale rigorous survey of sexual health behaviours and attitudes in Australia. It provides a benchmark of what Australians were like in 2002. Future generations will be able to look back at these data, and perhaps wonder why things were as they are now. For now, the findings provide an important reference point for people to make comparisons with their own behaviour. They also present general population averages that health care workers and sexual health professionals can use for comparison when dealing with patients and clients.

references and further reading

ACSF Investigators, 1992 'AIDS and sexual behaviour in France', *Nature* vol. 360, pp. 407–9.

Australian Bureau of Statistics 1995, *Demographic Estimates and Projections: Concepts, sources and methods (3228.0)*, Australian Government Publishing Service, Canberra.

Australian Bureau of Statistics 2003, *Marriages and Divorces, Australia, 2002 (3310.0)*, Australian Government Publishing Service, Canberra.

1: First times

Grunseit, A. and Richters, J. 2000, 'Age at first intercourse in an Australian national sample of technical college students', *Australian and New Zealand Journal of Public Health*, vol. 24, pp. 11–16.

Richters, J., Grunseit, A., Crawford, J., Song, A. and Kippax, S. (in press), 'Stability and change in sexual practices among first-year Australian university students 1990–1999', *Archives of Sexual Behavior*.

Rissel, C.E., Richters, J., Grulich, A.E., de Visser, R.O. and Smith, A.M.A. 2003, 'Sex in Australia: First experiences of vaginal intercourse and oral sex among a representative sample of adults', *Australian and New Zealand Journal of Public Health*, vol. 27, pp. 131–7.

Van de Ven, P., Rawstorne, P. and Treloar, C. (eds) 2002, *HIV/AIDS, Hepatitis C & Related Diseases in Australia: Annual report of behaviour 2002*, National Centre in HIV Social Research, Sydney.

2: What people do

Comfort, A. (ed.) 1972, *The Joy of Sex: A gourmet guide to love-making*, Rigby and Quartet Books, London.

De Visser, R.O., Smith, A.M.A., Rissel, C.E., Richters, J. and Grulich, A.E. 2003, 'Sex in Australia: Heterosexual experience and recent heterosexual encounters among a representative sample of adults', *Australian and New Zealand Journal of Public Health*, vol. 27, pp. 146–54.

Grulich, A.E., de Visser, R.O., Smith, A.M.A., Rissel, C.E. and Richters, J. 2003, 'Sex in Australia: Homosexual experience and recent homosexual encounters among a representative sample of adults', *Australian and New Zealand Journal of Public Health*, vol. 27, pp. 155–63.

Haavio-Mannila, E. and Kontula, O. 1997, 'Correlates of increased sexual satisfaction', *Archives of Sexual Behavior*, vol. 26, pp. 399–419.

Hite, S. 1976, *The Hite Report: A nationwide study of female sexuality*, Macmillan, New York.

Hubert, M., Bajos, N. and Sandfort, T. (eds) 1998, *Sexual Behaviour and HIV/AIDS in Europe*, UCL Press, London.

Richters, J., de Visser, R. and Rissel, C. 2004, 'Sexual practices at last heterosexual encounter and occurrence of orgasm', paper presented to ASSERT National Sexology Conference, Sydney, December.

Smith, G. 2001, 'Heterosexual and homosexual anal intercourse: An international perspective', *Venereology*, vol. 14, pp. 28–37.

Stone, H.M. and Stone, A. 1963, *A Marriage Manual: A practical guide-book to sex and marriage*, Angus & Robertson, Sydney (first published 1939).

Van de Velde, T.H. 1957, *Ideal Marriage: Its physiology and technique*, William Heinemann Medical Books, London.

3: How often

Richters, J., Grulich, A.E., de Visser, R.O., Smith, A.M.A. and Rissel, C.E. 2003, 'Sex in Australia: Sexual and emotional satisfaction and preferred frequency of sex among a representative sample of adults', *Australian and New Zealand Journal of Public Health*, vol. 27, pp. 171–9.

4: How many partners

Alexander, M.G. and Fisher, T.D. 2003, 'Truth and consequences: Using the bogus pipeline to examine sex differences in self-reported sexuality', *Journal of Sex Research*, vol. 40, pp. 27–35.

De Visser, R.O., Smith, A.M.A., Rissel, C.E., Richters, J. and Grulich, A.E. 2003, 'Sex in Australia: Heterosexual experience and recent heterosexual encounters among a representative sample of adults', *Australian and New Zealand Journal of Public Health*, vol. 27, pp. 146–54.

Grulich, A.E., de Visser, R.O., Smith, A.M.A., Rissel, C.E. and Richters, J. 2003, 'Sex in Australia: Homosexual experience and recent homosexual encounters among a representative sample of adults', *Australian and New Zealand Journal of Public Health*, vol. 27, pp. 155–63.

Hull, P., Van de Ven, P., Prestage, G., Rawstorne, P., Grulich, A., Crawford, J., Kippax, S., Madeddu, D., McGuigan, D. and Nicholas, A. 2003, *Gay Community Periodic Survey: Sydney 1996–2002*, Monograph 2/2003, National Centre in HIV Social Research, Sydney.

Johnson, A., Wadsworth, J., Wellings, K. and Field, J. 1994, *Sexual Attitudes and Lifestyles*, Blackwell, Oxford, pp. 203–8.

5: Attitudes towards sex

Australian Bureau of Statistics 1995, *Demographic Estimates and Projections: Concepts, sources and methods (3228.0)*, Australian Government Publishing Service, Canberra.

Australian Bureau of Statistics 2003, *Marriages and Divorces, Australia, 2002 (3310.0)*, Australian Government Publishing Service, Canberra.

Connell, R.W. 1995, *Masculinities*, Allen & Unwin, Sydney.

Herek, G.M. 2000 'Sexual prejudice and gender: Do heterosexuals' attitudes towards lesbians and gay men differ?' *Journal of Social Issues*, vol. 56, pp. 251–66.

Hopwood, M. and Connors, J. 2002, 'Heterosexual attitudes to homosexuality: Homophobia at a rural Australian university', in *From Here to Diversity: The social impact of lesbian and gay issues in education in Australia and New Zealand*, eds K.H. Robinson, J. Irwin and T. Ferfolja, Haworth Press, New York, pp. 79–94.

McKee, A. (Co-investigator), *Understanding Pornography in Australia* research project, Queensland University of Technology, personal communication, 23 February 2004.

Plummer, D.C. 2001, 'The quest for modern manhood: Masculine stereotypes, peer culture and the social significance of homophobia', *Journal of Adolescence*, vol. 24, pp. 15–23.

Richters, J. and Song, A. 1999, 'Australian university students agree with Clinton's definition of sex', *BMJ*, vol. 318, p. 1011.

Rissel, C.E., Richters, J., Grulich, A.E., de Visser, R.O. and Smith, A.M.A. 2003, 'Sex in Australia: Attitudes toward sex in a representative sample of adults', *Australian and New Zealand Journal of Public Health*, vol. 27, pp. 118–23.

Schmidt, G., Klusmann, D., Zeitschel, U. and Lange, C. 1994, 'Changes in adolescents' sexuality between 1970 and 1990 in West-Germany', *Archives of Sexual Behavior*, vol. 23, pp. 489–513.

6: Fun for one

Acker, E. 2001, 'Contradictory possibilities of cyberspace for generating romance', *Australian Journal of Communication*, vol. 28, pp. 103–16.

Allgeier, A.R. and Allgeier, E.R. 1995, *Sexual Interactions*, D.C. Heath, Lexington, MA.

Anonymous 2004, 'Learn how to make a perfect match click', *Daily Telegraph*, 27 January.

Bishop, C. and Osthelder, X. (eds) 2001, *Sexualia: From prehistory to cyberspace*, Könemann, Cologne.

Comfort, A. (ed.) 1972, *The Joy of Sex: A gourmet guide to lovemaking*, Rigby and Quartet Books, London.

Gregg, N. 2004, 'Cyber romance', *Courier-Mail*, 9 February.

Hillier, L., Kurdas, C. and Horsley, P. 2001, *'It's Just Easier': The Internet as a safety-net for same sex attracted young people*, Australian Research Centre in Sex, Health and Society, Melbourne.

Jackman, C. 2004, 'One man's online love story—lovers in the air', *Australian Magazine*, 14 February.

Leitenberg, H., Detzer, M.J. and Srebnik, D. 1993, 'Gender differences in masturbation and the relation of masturbation experience in preadolescence and/or early adolescence to sexual behavior and sexual adjustment in young adulthood', *Archives of Sexual Behavior*, vol. 22, pp. 87–98.

Manktelow, N. 2004, 'Love bytes', *Age*, 12 February.

Richters, J., Grulich, A.E., de Visser, R.O., Smith, A.M.A. and Rissel, C.E. 2003, 'Sex in Australia: Autoerotic, esoteric and other sexual practices engaged in by a representative sample of adults', *Australian and New Zealand Journal of Public Health*, vol. 27, pp. 180–90.

Silverstein, J. and Lasky, M. 2003, *Online Dating for Dummies*, John Wiley & Sons, New York.

Yavascaoglu, I., Oktay, B., Simsek, U., Ozyurt, M. 1999, 'Role of ejaculation in the treatment of chronic non-bacterial prostatitis', *International Journal of Urology*, vol. 6, pp. 130–4.

7: Kinky stuff

Agnew, J. 2001, 'An overview of paraphilia', *Venereology*, vol. 14, pp. 148–56.

Agnew, J. 2000, 'Anal manipulation as a source of sexual pleasure', *Venereology*, vol. 13, pp. 169–76.

American Psychiatric Association 2000, *Diagnostic and Statistical Manual of Mental Disorders: DSM-IV-TR*, 4th edn, text revision, APA, Washington, DC. Definition of paraphilias as quoted in Medline's Medical Subject Headings, at <www.ncbi.nlm.nih.gov/entrez/query.fcgi>, accessed 7 April 2004.

Bullough, V.L. 2001, 'Paraphilias: A response', *Venereology*, vol. 14, pp. 141–2.

Kinsey, A., Pomeroy, W. and Martin, C. 1948, *Sexual Behavior in the Human Male*, W.B. Saunders, Philadelphia.

Kippax, S., Campbell, D., Van de Ven, P., Crawford, J., Prestage, G. Knox, S. et al. 1998, 'Cultures of sexual adventurism as markers of HIV seroconversion: A case control study in a cohort of Sydney gay men', *AIDS Care*, vol. 10, pp. 677–88.

Love, B. 1992, *The Encyclopedia of Unusual Sex Practices*, Barricade Books, Fort Lee, NJ.

Richters, J., Grulich, A.E., de Visser, R.O., Smith, A.M.A. and Rissel, C.E. 2003, 'Sex in Australia: Esoteric and other sexual practices engaged in by a representative sample of adults', *Australian and New Zealand Journal of Public Health*, vol. 27, pp. 180–90.

8: Gay and straight

Hillier, L., Warr, D. and Haste, B. 1996, *The Rural Mural: Sexuality and diversity in rural youth*, Centre for the Study of Sexually Transmissible Diseases, Melbourne.

Johnson, A., Wadsworth, J., Wellings, K. and Field, J. 1994, *Sexual Attitudes and Lifestyles*, Blackwell, Oxford.

Johnson, A.M., Mercer, C.H., Erens, B., Copas, A.J., McManus, S., Wellings, K., Fenton, K.A., Korovessis, C., Macdowall, W., Nanchahal, K., Purdon, S. and Field, J. 2001, 'Sexual behaviour in Britain: Partnerships, practices, and HIV risk behaviours', *Lancet*, vol. 358, pp. 1835–42.

Kinsey, A.C., Pomeroy, W.B. and Martin, C.E. 1948, *Sexual Behavior in the Human Male*, W.B. Saunders, Philadelphia, p. 638.

Laumann, E.O., Gagnon, J.H., Michael, R.T. and Michaels, S. 1994, *The Social Organization of Sexuality: Sexual practices in the United States*, University of Chicago Press, Chicago.

Plummer, D.C., 2001, 'The quest for modern manhood: Masculine stereotypes, peer culture and the social significance of homophobia', *Journal of Adolescence*, vol. 24, pp. 15–23.

Richters, J. 1998, 'Understanding sexual orientation: A plea for clarity', *Reproductive Health Matters*, vol. 6, no. 12, pp. 144–9.

Smith, A.M.A., Rissel, C.E., Richters, J., Grulich, A.E. and de Visser, R.O. 2003, 'Sex in Australia: Sexual identity, sexual attraction, and sexual experience among a representative sample of adults', *Australian and New Zealand Journal of Public Health*, vol. 27, pp. 138–45.

9: Domestic bliss

Crawford, J., Kippax, S. and Waldby, C. 1994, 'Women's sex talk and men's sex talk: Different worlds', *Feminism & Psychology*, vol. 4, pp. 571–87.

Hollway, W. 1983, 'Heterosexual sex: Power and desire for the other', in *Sex & Love*, eds S. Cartledge and J. Ryan, Women's Press, London, pp. 124–40.

Richters, J., Grulich, A.E., de Visser, R.O., Smith, A.M.A. and Rissel, C.E. 2003, 'Sex in Australia: Sexual and emotional satisfaction in regular relationships and preferred frequency of sex among a representative sample of adults', *Australian and New Zealand Journal of Public Health*, vol. 27, pp. 171–9.

Rissel, C.E., Richters, J., Grulich, A.E., de Visser, R.O. and Smith, A.M.A. 2003, 'Sex in Australia: Selected characteristics of regular sexual relationships', *Australian and New Zealand Journal of Public Health*, vol. 27, pp. 124–30.

10: Is your partner cheating on you?

Rissel, C.E., Richters, J., Grulich, A.E., de Visser, R.O. and Smith, A.M.A. 2003a, 'Sex in Australia: Attitudes toward sex in a representative sample of adults', *Australian and New Zealand Journal of Public Health*, vol. 27, pp. 118–23.

Rissel, C.E., Richters, J., Grulich, A.E., de Visser, R.O. and Smith, A.M.A. 2003b, 'Sex in Australia: Selected characteristics of regular sexual relationships', *Australian and New Zealand Journal of Public Health*, vol. 27, pp. 124–30.

11: Getting pregnant

Australian Institute of Health and Welfare 1999, *Adoptions Australia 1997–1998*, AIHW cat. no. CWS–7, p. 6.

Cheesbrough, S., Ingham, R. and Massey, D. 1999, *Reducing the Rate of Teenage Conceptions. A review of the international evidence on preventing and reducing teenage conceptions: The United States, Canada, Australia and New Zealand*, Health Education Authority, London.

Darroch, J.E., Frost, J.J., Singh, S. and the study team, *Can More Progress Be Made? Teenage sexual and reproductive behavior in developed countries*, Alan Guttmacher Institute, New York. Available at <www.guttmacher.org>, accessed January 2004.

Rissel, C., Smith, A., Richters, J., Grulich, A. and de Visser, R. 2003, 'The Australian Study of Health and Relationships: Results for Central Sydney, Inner-Eastern Sydney, and New South Wales', *NSW Public Health Bulletin*, vol. 14, pp. 133–44.

Smith, A.M.A., Rissel, C.E., Richters, J., Grulich, A.E. and de Visser, R.O. 2003, 'Sex in Australia: Reproductive experiences and reproductive health among a representative sample of women', *Australian and New Zealand Journal of Public Health*, vol. 27, pp. 204–9.

12: Not getting pregnant

Hatcher, R.A., Trussell, J., Stewart, F., Stewart, G.K., Kowal, D., Guest, F., Cates, W. and Policar, M.S. 2000, *Contraceptive Technology*, BMJ Books, London.

Richters, J., Grulich, A.E., de Visser, R.O., Smith, A.M.A. and Rissel, C.E. 2003, 'Sex in Australia: Contraceptive practices among a representative sample of women', *Australian and New Zealand Journal of Public Health*, vol. 27, pp. 210–16.

Rissel, C.E., Richters, J., Grulich, A.E., de Visser, R.O. and Smith, A.M.A. 2003, 'Sex in Australia: Selected characteristics of regular sexual relationships', *Australian and New Zealand Journal of Public Health*, vol. 27, pp. 124–30.

Santow, G. 1991, 'Trends in contraception and sterilization in Australia', *Australian and New Zealand Journal of Obstetrics and Gynaecology*, vol. 31, pp. 201–8.

Smith, A., Agius, P., Dyson, S., Mitchell, A. and Pitts, M. 2003, *Secondary Students and Sexual Health 2002*, Australian Research Centre in Sex, Health and Society, Melbourne.

13: Sexual difficulties

Bittman, M. and Pixley, J. 1997, *The Double Life of the Family*, Allen & Unwin, Sydney.

Dempsey, K. 1997, *Inequalities in Marriage: Australia and beyond*, Oxford University Press, Melbourne.

Hawaleshka, D. 2003, 'Viagra's new competition', *Maclean's*, vol. 116, no. 50, 15 December, pp. 34–7, 38–41.

Hite, S. 1976, *The Hite Report: A nationwide study of female sexuality*, Macmillan, New York.

Kaschak, E. and Tiefer, L. (eds) 2001, *A New View of Women's Sexual Problems*, Haworth, New York.

Kitzinger, S. 1983, *Woman's Experience of Sex*, Dorling Kindersley, London.

Laumann, E.O., Paik, A. and Rosen, R.C. 1999, 'Sexual dysfunction in the United States: Prevalence and predictors', *JAMA*, vol. 281, pp. 537–44.

Morrow, R. 1994, 'The sexological construction of sexual dysfunction', *Australian and New Zealand Journal of Sociology*, vol. 30, pp. 20–35.

Pfizer, information about Viagra (sildenafil citrate), at <www.viagra.com>, accessed 21 January 2004.

Richters, J., Grulich, A.E., de Visser, R.O., Smith, A.M.A. and Rissel, C.E. 2003, 'Sex in Australia: Sexual difficulties in a representative sample of adults', *Australian and New Zealand Journal of Public Health* vol. 27, pp. 164–70.

Steffens, M. 2003, 'Not just a headache, darling', ABC Website 7 August 2003, available at <www.abc.net.au/health/features/headache/default.htm>, accessed 20 January 2004.

14: Sexual assault

David, T. and Lee, C. 1996, 'Sexual assault: Myths and stereotypes among Australian adolescents', *Sex Roles*, vol. 34, pp. 787–803.

De Visser, R.O., Smith, A.M.A., Rissel, C.E., Richters, J. and Grulich, A.E., 2003 'Sex in Australia: Experiences of sexual coercion among a representative sample of adults', *Australian and New Zealand Journal of Public Health* vol. 27, pp. 198–203.

Heilpern, D.M. 1998, *Fear or Favour: Sexual assault of young prisoners*, Southern Cross University Press, Lismore, NSW.

Laumann, E.O., Gagnon, J.H., Michael, R. and Michaels, S. 1994, *The Social Organization of Sexuality: Sexual practices in the United States*, University of Chicago Press, Chicago.

Moreton, R. 2003, 'A focus group study of young women's perceptions of risk and behaviours', *Youth Studies Australia*, vol. 22, no. 3, pp. 18–24.

Xenos, S. and Smith, D. 2001, 'Perceptions of rape and sexual assault among Australian adolescents and young adults', *Journal of Interpersonal Violence*, vol. 16, pp. 1103–19.

15: Paying for sex
Harcourt, C. and Donovan, B. 2000, *The Health & Welfare Needs of Female & Transgender Street-Based Sex Workers in New South Wales*, State Health Publication No. (AIDS) 990187, NSW Health Department, Sydney.

Richters, J., Donovan, B., Gerofi, J. and Watson, L. 1988, 'Low condom breakage rate in commercial sex' [letter], *Lancet*, vol. 2, no. 8626–8627, pp. 1487–8.

Rissel, C.E., Richters, J., Grulich, A.E., de Visser, R.O. and Smith, A.M.A. 2003, 'Sex in Australia: Experiences of commercial sex in a representative sample of adults', *Australian and New Zealand Journal of Public Health*, vol. 27, pp. 191–7.

16: Sexually transmitted infections and safe sex
Cowan, F.M., Copas, A., Johnson, A.M., Ashley, R., Corey, L. and Mindel, A. 2002, 'Herpes simplex virus type 1 infection: A sexually transmitted infection of adolescence?', *Sexually Transmitted Infections*, vol. 78, pp. 346–8.

De Visser, R.O., Smith, A.M.A., Rissel, C.E., Richters, J. and Grulich, A.E. 2003, 'Sex in Australia: Safer sex and condom use among a representative sample of adults', *Australian and New Zealand Journal of Public Health*, vol. 27, pp. 223–9.

Grulich, A.E., de Visser, R.O., Smith, A.M.A., Rissel, C.E. and Richters, J. 2003a, 'Sex in Australia: Knowledge about sexually transmitted infections among a representative sample of adults', *Australian and New Zealand Journal of Public Health*, vol. 27, pp. 230–3.

Grulich, A.E., de Visser, R.O., Smith, A.M.A., Rissel, C.E. and Richters, J. 2003b, 'Sex in Australia: Sexually transmissible infection and blood-borne virus history in a representative sample of adults', *Australian and New Zealand Journal of Public Health*, vol. 27, pp. 234–41.

International Collaboration on HIV Optimism 2003, 'HIV treatments optimism among gay men: An international perspective', *Journal of Acquired Immune Deficiency Syndromes*, vol. 32, pp. 545–50.

Mindel, A. 1998, 'Genital herpes—how much of a public-health problem?', *Lancet*, vol. 351 (supplement III), pp. 16–18.

National Centre in HIV Epidemiology and Clinical Research 2003, *HIV/AIDS, Viral Hepatitis and Sexually Transmissible Infections in Australia: Annual surveillance report 2003*, NCHECR, Sydney.

NSW Health 2003, 'HIV plan aims to stop infection increase' [media release], 17 November, Sydney.

Rogow, D. and Horowitz, S. 1995, 'Withdrawal: A review of the literature and an agenda for research', *Studies in Family Planning*, vol. 26, pp. 140–53.

Tideman, R.L., Taylor, J., Marks, C., Seifert, C., Berry, G., Trudinger, B., Cunningham, A. and Mindel, A. 2001, 'Sexual and demographic risk factors for herpes simplex type 1 and 2 in women attending an antenatal clinic', *Sexually Transmitted Infections*, vol. 77, pp. 413–15.

Qld Health Youth Site: Sexual Health, HIV/AIDS and Hepatitis C at <http://www.health.qld.gov.au/istaysafe/default.asp>

*my*Dr: Sexual Health Centre at <http://www.mydr.com.au/default.asp?Section=sexualhealth>

NSW Health: Sexually Transmitted Diseases and their Prevention at <http://www.health.nsw.gov.au/health-public-affairs/publications/std/>

Better Health Channel: STDs at <http://www.betterhealth.vic.gov.au/>

Sexual Health and Family Planning Australia: Contacts in all states at <http://www.fpa.net.au/links.htm>

FPA Healthrites (mail-order publications), telephone: (02) 8752 4307, fax: (02) 9799 8835, email: healthrites@fpahealth.org.au

17: Sex in Australia

ACSF Investigators, 1992 'AIDS and sexual behaviour in France', *Nature* vol. 360, pp. 407–9.

Johnson, A., Wadsworth, J., Wellings, K. and Field, J. 1994, *Sexual Attitudes and Lifestyles*, Blackwell, Oxford.

Johnson, A.M., Mercer, C.H., Erens, B., Copas, A.J., McManus, S., Wellings, K., Fenton, K.A., Korovessis, C., Macdowall, W., Nanchahal, K., Purdon, S. and Field, J. 2001, 'Sexual behaviour in Britain: Partnerships, practices, and HIV risk behaviours', *Lancet*, vol. 358, pp. 1835–42.

Laumann, E.O., Gagnon, J.H., Michael, R.T. and Michaels, S. 1994, *The Social Organization of Sexuality: Sexual practices in the United States*, University of Chicago Press, Chicago.

Leridon, H., van Zessen, G. and Hubert, M. 1998, 'The Europeans and their sexual partners' in *Sexual Behaviour and HIV/AIDS in Europe*, eds M. Hubert, N. Bajos and T. Sandfort, UCL Press, London, pp. 165–96.

Appendix 1: The survey

Blewett, N. 2003, *AIDS in Australia: the primitive years. Reflections on Australia's policy response to the AIDS epidemic*, Australian Health Policy Institute, University of Sydney, Sydney.

Brewer, D.D., Potterat, J.J., Garrett, S.B., Muth, S.Q., Roberts, J.M., Jr, Kasprzyk, D., Montano, D.E. and Darrow, W.W. 2000, 'Prostitution and the sex discrepancy in reported number of sexual partners', *Proceedings of the National Academy of Sciences of the United States of America*, vol. 97, pp. 12 385–8.

Brown, N.R. and Sinclair, R.C. 1999, 'Estimating number of lifetime sexual partners: Men and women do it differently', *Journal of Sex Research*, vol. 36, pp. 292–7.

Crawford, J., Kippax, S., Rodden, P., Donohoe, S. and Van de Ven, P. 1998, *Male Call 96: National telephone survey of men who have sex with men*, National Centre in HIV Social Research, Sydney.

Dunne, M. 1998, 'Sex surveys: What does it mean when thirty to forty percent don't participate?' *Venereology*, vol. 11, no. 2, pp. 33–7.

Eriksen, J. and Steffen, S. 1999, *Kiss and Tell: Surveying sex in the twentieth century*, Harvard University Press, Cambridge, MA.

Hite, S. 1976, *The Hite Report: A nationwide study of female sexuality*, Macmillan, New York.

Johnson, A., Wadsworth, J., Wellings, K. and Field, J. 1994, *Sexual Attitudes and Lifestyles*, Blackwell, Oxford.

Johnson, A.M., Mercer, C.H., Erens, B., Copas, A.J., McManus, S., Wellings, K., Fenton, K.A., Korovessis, C., Macdowall, W., Nanchahal, K., Purdon, S. and Field, J. 2001, 'Sexual behaviour in Britain: Partnerships, practices, and HIV risk behaviours', *Lancet*, vol. 358, pp. 1835–42.

Kinsey, A., Pomeroy, W. and Martin, C. 1948, *Sexual Behavior in the Human Male*, W.B. Saunders, Philadelphia.

Kinsey, A., Pomeroy, W., Martin, C. and Gebhard, P. 1953, *Sexual Behavior in the Human Female*, W.B. Saunders, Philadelphia.

Laumann, E.O., Gagnon, J.H., Michael, R.T. and Michaels, S. 1994, *The Social Organization of Sexuality: Sexual practices in the United States*, University of Chicago Press, Chicago.

Laumann, E.O., Michael, R.T. and Gagnon, J.H. 1994, 'A political history of the National Sex Survey of Adults', *Family Planning Perspectives*, vol. 26, no. 1, pp. 34–8.

Masters, W.H. and Johnson, V.E. 1966, *Human Sexual Response*, Little, Brown, Boston.

Smith, A.M.A., Rissel, C.E., Richters, J., Grulich, A.E. and de Visser, R.O. 2003, 'Sex in Australia: A guide for readers', *Australian and New Zealand Journal of Public Health*, vol. 27, pp. 103–5.

Smith, A.M.A., Rissel, C.E., Richters, J., Grulich, A.E. and de Visser, R.O. 2003, 'Sex in Australia: The rationale and methods of the Australian Study of Health and Relationships', *Australian and New Zealand Journal of Public Health*, vol. 27, pp. 106–17.

Williamson, M., Baker, D. and Jorm, L. 2001, 'The NSW Health Survey Program: Overview and methods, 1996–2000', *NSW Public Health Bulletin*, vol. 12, no. S-2.

appendix 1: the survey

Researching sex

Most people acquire their knowledge about sex—especially the 'how to' variety—from articles in magazines. Some journalists thoroughly research their topic and base what they say on scientific findings, but short deadlines and production pressures can mean a journalist only has time to ask a few friends about their experiences. The resulting information can be quite unreliable.

Magazines also often present the results of reader surveys. These are based on questionnaires in magazines that readers fill in and send back to the magazine's editors. Obviously, only certain types of people buy any particular magazine, and only a small subset of these readers return the questionnaires. At best, the results might be typical of the average readers of that magazine (or the more sexually interested ones), but they could never be claimed as representative of the general population. In any case, the questions are often so loosely worded that it's not at all clear what the readers' answers mean.

Other large surveys are done by researchers or writers who place advertisements and send out letters asking people to volunteer to be part of the survey. The very influential *Hite Report* on women's sexuality (published in 1976) is an example of this sort of work. Because people write in their own words in answer to open-ended questions, such surveys give an insight into individual men's and women's thoughts and feelings. But because the respondents choose to be part of the survey (perhaps because they particularly like the researcher's point of view or because they feel strongly about something in the study, such as childhood sexual abuse), such surveys are not representative of the population in general. We will never know whether the women who answered Shere Hite's questionnaires were typical of American women at the time or not.

Until the advent of AIDS in the 1980s, the most substantial source of information about sex was from the pioneer sex researchers Alfred Kinsey and his team. Dr Kinsey's group interviewed thousands of men and women in the United States during the 1940s and 1950s. The respondents were not randomly selected, as is the case in a modern survey, and Kinsey has been criticised for this—perhaps unfairly, as it would not have been possible to do otherwise at the time. However, rather than using volunteers who select themselves, Kinsey preferred to get permission to interview all the members of groups such as sporting clubs or all the staff of a firm, to get an unbiased picture. A huge range of people were studied, including university students and military personnel. The huge scholarly tomes that reported the research became best-sellers, so anxious were people to find out about what other people did in those days when sex was not openly discussed.

Until the advent of AIDS in the 1980s, the most substantial source of information about sex was from the pioneer sex researchers Alfred Kinsey and his team.

In the 1960s, the sex therapist team of Dr William Masters and Virginia Johnson closely studied friends and associates while they had sex in the laboratory. This research revealed much about the human physiological response during sex and provided new insights into human sexuality—confirming, for example, the importance of clitoral stimulation for women. However, the research suffered from a major drawback. Masters and Johnson assumed that the ability to have an orgasm during intercourse was the criterion for adequate sexual function. They then selected couples who could do this for their studies in the laboratory. The volunteers had to be able to have sex in front of researchers while having their heartbeat and other physiological responses measured. Such couples were not likely to be typical of ordinary people having sex. Indeed, Shere Hite's later published findings that only around 30 per cent of her 3000 respondents regularly reached orgasm from intercourse dramatically questioned Masters and Johnson's assumption that women who did not reach orgasm from intercourse were a dysfunctional minority. Nonetheless, Masters and Johnson's work had a huge influence on the training of sex counsellors and therapists in North America and around the world.

Counsellors and sex therapists are another source of information about sex and relationships. Their knowledge is generally based on clinical experience. Some counsellors see thousands of clients in the course of their careers and often have good insights into sex and relationship issues. However, therapists and counsellors see people with problems and do not see the majority of people who do not have a problem. Nor do they see people who have a problem but do not go to a professional for help.

When AIDS appeared in the early 1980s, doctors studying the epidemic asked new questions about sexual behaviour. In order to calculate how fast the new disease might spread, they needed to know how often people had intercourse (or other sexual practices that could pass on the disease) and how many partners they had. They asked what percentage of the population had same-sex partners. Today these seem simple questions, but at the time we did not know the answers. Thus for the first time, health authorities became interested in spending money on large national surveys about sexual behaviour.

During the 1960s and 1970s, at the same time as the rise of sex therapy, social scientists started to study sex in the same way as other social behaviour. In the 1980s and 1990s, they teamed up with epidemiologists to do national representative sex surveys. Despite some opposition, surveys were done in the United States and in the United Kingdom around 1990.

The Australian Study of Health and Relationships

When we started to develop our Australian survey in the late 1990s, we were fortunate to have the American and British household surveys to draw upon, as well as telephone surveys from France, New Zealand and elsewhere. We used or adapted questions from their questionnaires and at times we learnt from their mistakes. In doing so, we drew on the experience that we and our colleagues had gained through two decades of work in public health, sexual health, family planning and HIV prevention.

Telephone interviews were conducted with 19 307 randomly selected people aged over sixteen and under sixty from households in all states and territories. It took a team of specially trained interviewers from mid-2001 to mid-2002 to complete all the interviews. A total of 111 290 telephone calls were made to achieve this. Of those people contacted who were eligible to take part, 73 per cent agreed to do so (69 per cent of men and 78 per cent of women). In some areas and age groups, response rates were slightly lower or higher than this average. For example, people living in cities are less keen on responding to surveys than country people, and people in their twenties are less likely to respond than older people. So that the published results would be reliably representative of the population as a whole, statistical adjustments were made to the figures to allow for these variations in response rates by location, age and sex.

After these adjustments were made, the sample was largely typical of Australians, but there were some differences when compared to the Census. Our respondents were more likely to say they had no religion than people responding to the Census. This may be because the Census (a written questionnaire) asks 'What is the person's religion?' and offers a series of religions as possible responses, with the response 'No religion' tucked down at the bottom of the section under the space marked 'Other— please specify'. People answering the Census may not notice that 'No religion' is an option. Possibly they may feel that as the Census form is a government document they should state their 'official' religion, for example the one in which they were baptised, even if they do not currently practise it. Our interviewers asked 'Do you have a particular religion or faith?' and only asked what it was if people said 'yes'. This made it very easy for people to say 'no'.

Our respondents also reported higher incomes than those completing the Census form. This might be related to the fact that our survey was anonymous and independent of the government, so people had no reason to fear the information would be passed to the Tax Office. It may also be that people overstated their incomes to us to make themselves sound more successful (researchers call this 'social desirability bias'). Further details about how the sample of people for this survey was selected can be found in Appendix 2: People in the survey.

The Australian Study of Health and Relationships was funded by the Australian Government. Initially the research team, led by Dr Chris Rissel and Associate Professor Anthony Smith, applied for funding from the National Health and Medical Research Council for a national sex survey and were successful in gaining support for a pilot test in New South Wales. No political objections were raised. It was treated like any other scientific study applying for funding. The main national study was funded directly by the Department of Health and Aged Care, with some state health departments also supporting the project. The federal government appointed an advisory committee of research experts to advise the project, but at no time was there any political attempt to stifle any aspect of the research, as had happened to earlier surveys in the United States and Britain. We like to think the fact that there were no substantial political barriers to our survey says something about straightforward Australian attitudes to sex.

The political context of the study

Australia had distinguished itself fifteen years earlier by responding to the AIDS epidemic with a bipartisan approach involving a partnership between affected people—mostly gay men—and researchers, governments and health services. The *Grim Reaper* advertising campaign and the huge media coverage in the 1980s meant that virtually every Australian had heard of AIDS. Australians soon became comfortable with using such words as 'condom' in conversation. Rarely were arguments about 'decency' used to prevent frank and open discussion of how HIV (the AIDS virus) was transmitted.

Although the Queensland state government did prohibit some educational campaigns—such as the proposed 'Bubble Boy' collector cards containing safe sex information for gay men, which it was feared would be attractive to under-age card collectors—by and large Australian governments have left educational and service organisations to get on with the job of providing the kind of safe sex material that works. For example, sexually explicit educational leaflets and advertisements are available for gay men and for sex workers. In response to the recent increases in HIV infections health educators are again visiting gay clubs, pubs and saunas to distribute health information.

Australians are fortunate that here, unlike in many other parts of the world, political schisms between conservative religious groups and the secular left are less pronounced. Although there is some controversy on sexual issues, sex is not a major topic of political debate. Health care services (including pregnancy termination and sexually transmitted disease clinics) and health educators (in schools and among high-risk groups) are largely left to get on with the job.

This generally calm atmosphere in relation to sex was reflected in the responses to our survey, both during its execution and when the main report was published. During the development of the survey and while the interviews were being conducted, we were approached on several occasions by interested journalists. We told them that although we were happy to answer questions and the survey was not a secret, we were not keen to publicise it actively as this would raise the risk of people making spoof calls. We did not want a rash of people (most likely men or teenagers) making telephone calls, pretending to be from the survey and asking people (most likely women) about their sexual practices. The journalists understood this and agreed to contact us when the results were available.

When the report was published as a series of articles in the *Australian and New Zealand Journal of Public Health* in April 2003, we had a launch in Melbourne to which the media were invited. We distributed a four-page summary of the findings. Newspaper, radio and television coverage of the study was nearly all positive. The few objections, made by people who rang radio stations or wrote letters to newspapers, were not about the survey or any of its findings. They were about the obvious policy recommendation arising from the finding that the typical age at first intercourse has gone down. We suggested that sex education should be given earlier, even to primary school pupils. This would mean that students would receive sex education before they become sexually active rather than afterwards.

Do people tell the truth in a sex survey?

A very common question about surveys of sexual behaviour is whether participants tell the truth. There is no 'gold standard' or perfect way to assess this. However, many studies have found what appears to be either a small under-reporting or some slight over-reporting of risky behaviours, with the general conclusion that most people tell the truth most of the time. What questions are asked and the way they are asked can influence the sort of replies that are given.

An enormous amount of effort in the Australian Study of Health and Relationships went into carefully framing questions about sexual behaviour in a way that gave the participant no reason to lie. Before the interviews began, we reviewed the questions asked in sex surveys in other countries to identify the most comprehensible, valid and reliable questions. All the interviewers underwent two days of training on sexual attitudes and what the final list of questions was designed to address. This was important, because the interviewer had to be non-judgmental about what a participant might say, even if the interviewer did not personally approve of it.

All the interviewers chose to work on this project: they were free to join other research projects. They were all highly experienced telephone interviewers who had worked on other health surveys, and this certainly contributed to the survey's excellent response rate of 73 per cent. All the interviewers were women, and although a male interviewer was available in case a participant asked to speak to a man, no-one took up the option.

The questions were asked in a professional, even clinical, manner so that the interview would seem practical and straight-forward—like going to the doctor and giving a medical history—and not prurient. Although some participants tried to joke or flirt with the interviewer, this was discouraged because the interviewer was simply trying to get an accurate answer, not to make friends with the participant. Feedback from a small proportion of participants who were rung twice for quality control purposes spoke very highly of the professionalism of the interviewers.

The interviews were conducted from a computer-based questionnaire using a system called CATI (computer-assisted telephone interview). Interviewers read out the questions as they appeared on the screen and then entered a number which corresponded to the response. The structured nature of the questions, with numbered answers, meant that participants at home did not have to verbally describe their sexual history, which could have been embarrassing if they were in the lounge room with the family listening in.

Considerable effort went into designing this CATI procedure. It had to accommodate the complete spectrum of possible responses—the respondent might be a 16-year-old virgin, a 34-year-old male sex worker, or a middle-aged married woman having a lesbian affair. The CATI program allows some sections to be skipped if they do not apply to a participant, and also to tailor questions. For example, if a man said that the last time he had sex was with a man, then further questions on the computer screen about this partner used the pronoun 'he' rather than 'she'. In the abbreviated version of the question-naire reproduced in Appendix 3, some of these variants are omitted or shown in square brackets.

Because there is so much boasting, joking, tale-telling—and keeping silent—around sex, it is suspected that respondents to sex surveys are unlikely to tell the truth about what they really

The respondent might be a 16-year-old virgin, a 34-year-old male sex worker, or a middle-aged married woman having a lesbian affair.

do. In fact, it seems from decades of research that sex is no more difficult to research accurately than other topics such as food and exercise. All surveys are affected by how people like to make themselves sound good in a conversation with an interviewer. Much of the skill and experience that goes into designing good interview questions is aimed at reducing this 'social desirability' factor and getting answers that are as accurate as possible.

Despite our best efforts, one area where social desirability does seem to affect responses is that men report having more sex, and more partners, than women do. Yet in a closed population of heterosexuals, the number of partners men have should equal the numbers women have. Various explanations have been suggested for this discrepancy, which turns up in almost all surveys. One is that the population is not closed: perhaps more men have sex with women overseas. Another is that because the age limits for our sample are the same for men and women, but many men have partners younger than themselves, some men report encounters with girls under sixteen. Conversely, older women in the sample may have partners over 60 (or no partners at all). Thus the average man aged 16–59 has more sex than the average woman aged 16–59. It has also been suggested that men visiting sex workers would account for the difference in reported numbers of partners, if men included sex workers when reporting how many women they had sex with. If women who do sex work are less likely to agree to take part in the survey, or are left out because they are not at home to answer the telephone, their male partners would not be recorded. This could also happen if women who do sex work do not count men who pay them as 'sexual partners' (and we know this is sometimes the case). We are inclined to think, however, that the main reason for the difference is that men like to show off about how much sex they have had, but many women are still worried that people will consider them 'sluts' if they have casual sex, or sex with too many men ('Now you'll think I'm awful'). This is discussed further in Chapter 4, 'How many partners'.

Although survey respondents may exaggerate or minimise some things, people are not usually very good at sustained lying. Even when talking to a stranger on the telephone, most people give a reasonably consistent story about themselves. The easiest way to do this is to tell the truth, more or less. The average person can easily 'omit' something from their history in an interview if it is something they usually do not talk about or something that does not fit into the image they have of themselves and usually present to others. A woman who gave up a baby for adoption when she was in her teens in the 1970s may omit to mention this to an interviewer, just as she may even have concealed the information from her own husband and children and friends ever since. A married man who occasionally meets other men for sex in the park but never talks about this and has no gay friends may 'forget' this when reporting his sexual partners in an interview. Survey researchers cannot do anything about this. In the end, an interview is just a conversation between two people, albeit a carefully scripted one for the interviewer. Nonetheless, it can also happen that an anonymous interview is the first opportunity in many years that a person has to tell their truth, their story, to say things that are not acceptable in ordinary social interaction. In an interview every response is valid, and there should be no judgment. So sometimes people tell of events—sexual assault, or an abortion, or underage sex—that they have never told anyone else.

As one measure of how truthful people had been, we asked them how embarrassing they had found the questionnaire. Overall about 6 per cent of men and 10 per cent of women said they had felt quite, very or extremely embarrassed—or to put it the other way round, more than 90 per cent of participants were not embarrassed at all or only slightly. Older participants were generally less embarrassed than younger participants.

The results of this sex survey are as accurate as the best surveys on other topics such as health behaviour, and better than any information we have had in the past about the sexual lives of Australians.

appendix 2: people in the survey

How the sample was chosen

We started off by discussing how best to conduct a national sex survey and then decided upon a telephone survey. Alternative methods, such as written questionnaires as part of a postal survey, or face-to-face interviews, have some major drawbacks for this type of research. Written questionnaires are cheaper to conduct, but many people who receive a printed questionnaire simply bin it or leave it lying round and forget to send it back, which makes the sample less typical of the population as a whole. Those who do reply tend to be more interested in the topic of the survey and better than average at reading and writing. This means that some people, such as migrants from non-English-speaking countries and those with little education, are less likely to be included.

Face-to-face interviews provide good quality data, but it would have been prohibitively expensive to randomly select nearly 20 000 people across Australia and then interview them in their homes. By comparison, telephone surveys are less expensive than face-to-face surveys, have adequate response rates, do not require high levels of literacy, can be highly structured and can provide good quality data. As well, nearly all Australian households (97 per cent) have at least one telephone.

Random selection

We then used a two-stage system to randomly select the people we asked to participate in the study. The first stage was working out which households we should phone. To begin with, we used the electronic White Pages telephone directory and a computer algorithm to identify the range of telephone numbers allocated to residential households. This was done to make the next step more efficient: computer-generating thousands of random phone numbers within that range. Based on previous research by the NSW Health Survey program, we knew that on average we needed to call six phone numbers to achieve one complete interview. As we were aiming for 20 000 interviews, we had to have over 120 000 telephone numbers.

Once we had a genuinely random list of telephone numbers to call, the second stage—obtaining participants—was to call each number to find out whether there were any people in the household who were eligible to take part in the survey. We were looking for people aged at least sixteen and under sixty years old. On average, each household was called up to six times to try and catch someone at home.

For the men's version of the survey, the process began with the interviewer briefly explaining she was conducting the Australian Study of Men's Health and Relationships, and asking whether there were any men in the household aged sixteen to fifty-nine. Depending on how many there were, one of them was chosen at random. For example, if there were three eligible men—Alan, Bill and Colin—their first names were typed in and then a number between 1 and 3 was randomly generated by the computer. If the number was 1, the interviewer would ask to speak with Alan. Only the selected respondent could be interviewed—it was not permissible to speak to Bill instead just because he happened to be available. Up to five attempts would be made to speak to Alan at a time convenient for him. The same principle was used for the women's survey.

Response rate and sample size

Overall, the response rate to the survey was a very acceptable 73 per cent. This compares well to the two large sexual health surveys conducted in Britain in 1990–91 and 2000, where the response rate was around 60 to 65 per cent. Women are generally more willing to respond to surveys than men, and our survey was no exception: the women's response rate was 78 per cent and the men's 69 per cent.

Across Australia, 19 307 interviews were conducted. Such a large number of people was needed so we could measure accurately how frequently some less common behaviours and practices occurred. For example, one estimate from the United States of the proportion of men who have ever had sex with another male was 4 per cent. In order to have a statistically precise estimate of this proportion of the population, about

400 men engaging in this behaviour are needed. Therefore if the real proportion of men who have ever had sex with men is 4 per cent, then 10 000 men overall are needed to end up with 400 men who have sex with men. The total number of participants needs to be doubled to allow for a similar calculation for women.

Who is missing?

No survey can include everyone. The Australian Study of Health and Relationships omitted:
- children and teenagers under sixteen
- people over sixty
- people without telephones
- people who don't live in households—for example those on oil rigs, in hostels or dormitories, in prison, in hospital, at boarding school or in university colleges
- people who refuse to answer surveys.

People who refuse to take part

Even though we made small adjustments in the figures to allow for the fact that women are more willing to take part in surveys, and for the higher and lower response rates in some geographic areas and among some age groups, a sample can never be perfectly typical of the population it is drawn from. Some people may simply refuse to take part in ways directly related to the topic of the survey. People who are uninterested in sex or who morally disapprove of it, except for making babies, are more likely to refuse. Research has also shown that people who are more sex-positive and have had more sexual experience are more likely to respond to surveys specifically concerning sex. Thus it is possible that our final estimates of the proportion of people who have more adventurous sex lives may be slightly exaggerated. On the other hand, there may be people who agreed to answer our questions but were unwilling to tell us about activities they regarded as shameful or kinky. We cannot tell to what extent one effect compensates for the other. It is likely, however, that there are more virgins among those who refused to participate than among those who took part. Despite our attempts to stress to people that we wanted to include everyone, adults who have never had a girlfriend or boyfriend may be embarrassed about this and decline to take part as soon as they hear the word 'relationships' in the interviewer's introduction to the survey.

People from different ethnic backgrounds

If you are gay, you may be disappointed that so much of the book is concerned with heterosexuals. The reason for this is that despite the large number of participants in the survey (19 307), only 156 men (1.6 per cent) think of themselves as gay and 77 women (0.8 per cent) think of themselves as lesbians. If you divide this group further into age groups, those with and without partners and so on, you end up with such tiny numbers in each category that the comparisons become unreliable. The main value of this study for research into the sexual and health concerns of homosexual and bisexual people is that the sample is representative, so we can compare it with other studies where large numbers of gay and bisexual people volunteer to take part.

People who could not speak English well were not included in the survey, because we could not afford to have the huge questionnaire translated into other languages and employ and train foreign-language interviewers. No single non-English-speaking ethnic group constitutes more than 2 per cent of the population. We have not been able to analyse whether people from different ethnic backgrounds who did take part in the survey, or indigenous Australians, have different sexual behaviour or attitudes. In the book we have sometimes noted that people from non-English-speaking backgrounds are different in some way (for example, they are on average less liberal in their sexual attitudes). This rather unsatisfactory category lumps Italians and Chinese, Pacific Islanders and South Americans together, but the findings may point to areas in which surveys in specific ethnic communities are needed. Already a team in Sydney has used our questionnaire as the basis for a telephone survey of Vietnamese Australians, and we hope this will be done for other language groups to identify any special sexual health needs.

Gays and lesbians?

We explained in Chapter 8, 'Gay and straight', that we believe our estimates for the proportion of gay men and lesbians nationally are correct—we don't think that gay people have been underrepresented in the survey.

Transgender and intersex people

Throughout this book we talked about men and women as if all human beings fell neatly into these categories. This is not true: in every society there are some people who do not conform to gender norms. Some babies are born with various kinds of intersex conditions. For example, a genetic male with XY chromosomes might have genitals that are female or ambiguous in appearance (what was previously called hermaphroditism). Some people born with features of both sexes have surgery during infancy and/or after puberty to 'correct' their appearance to that of either male or female. There are also people who—while their genetic make-up and physical features seem to match—are convinced they are living in the 'wrong' body. Many such people seek sex reassignment surgery to align their bodies with their internal sense of who they are. Others live as the other sex, either for brief periods or most of their lives, without having surgery. And there are other transgender people who do not seek to change themselves from one sex to the other but who feel that society is restrictive and wrong in requiring people to belong to only one sex and to conform to the 'rules' of appropriate gender behaviour.

Many people find behaviour that transgresses gender norms to be very offensive. Transgender people suffer a huge amount of prejudice and hostility unless they are transsexuals who can successfully 'pass' as members of their preferred gender.

Estimates based on reports of infants born with congenital conditions, surgery records, membership of transgender organisations and studies of transsexual and transgender volunteers suggest that about one person in 1000 has a transgender or intersex condition. If this is correct, the survey should have included about twenty transgender or intersex people, as long as they were not more likely to refuse the interview than other people. We would very much have liked to check this estimate from the survey data. However, the way we did the sampling made it very difficult to interview transgender and intersex people. Because most people are more willing to respond to a survey that is specific to their own sex, the study was done using separate samples of men and women. The interviewers rang each household and said, 'First I need to confirm that you are a woman aged between sixteen and fifty-nine' (or the equivalent for the men's survey). This made it very hard for transgender people to be interviewed unless they 'outed' themselves by directly telling the interviewer that they were (for example) a woman who was born a man.

We had prepared special versions of the questionnaire to suit people in this situation (for example not assuming that all women had vaginas, and adding extra questions about whether they had had sex reassignment or 'correction' surgery for intersex conditions), but the special questions were never used. Understandably, any transgender or intersex people who were rung by our interviewers either refused to respond to the survey or gave answers simply as men or women, saying nothing about their status or medical history.

People over sixty

The study has been criticised for leaving out older people. This is not because we think sexual life is over at sixty—it's not. The idea that older people are no longer interested in 'that sort of thing' is dying out. Although older people are more likely to have health problems or sexual difficulties that interfere with having intercourse, the retirement years can be a very happy time for a sexual relationship. On the other hand, more people, especially women, find themselves without partners as they age, which makes it increasingly difficult for them to have an active sex life. But some people do find new partners and new happiness in their sexual lives. The main reason for leaving older people out of the survey was not because their sexual lives don't exist or don't matter, but because the survey was funded with health care dollars.

Our brief was to obtain as much data as possible on groups of people whose sexual health is at particular risk: those who risk unwanted pregnancy or sexually transmitted diseases. Some state health departments gave us additional funding to add particular 'risk groups' to the sample, such as men in parts of central Sydney. (We adjusted the figures during our analysis to allow for these respondents, so that the final results were not skewed.) People over sixty do not get pregnant, and they very rarely catch sexual infections. They very rarely get sexually assaulted, and they don't often visit sex workers. Although it would have been very interesting for us to compare their sexual attitudes with those of younger people, we could not justify the cost of interviewing people aged sixty and over. We very much hope that another team will explore these issues in a survey of older people. Ideally such a survey should collect more detail than we did about health problems and health care, so that we can learn how best to ensure long and happy sexual lives for all our citizens.

appendix 3: the questionnaire

This is a simplified and edited version of the questionnaire computer program used for the survey—skips and filters are not shown. Not all the questions shown were asked of all the respondents. This one is based on the women's questionnaire, with questions on the men's version shown in some places for clarity, but not all the variants are shown. In the variant questions, wording was adjusted according to whether the respondent was a man or a woman and whether the partner referred to was male or female, regular or non-regular (casual). Response options are not shown where questions invited a simple yes/no response or a number (such as number of sexual partners). 'Don't know' and 'Refused' response options are generally not shown.

Roman print in square brackets is used for alternative or additional wording used where appropriate according to the gender of the respondent or the answers to previous questions. It shows words actually read out by interviewers. Italic print in square brackets is used for (1) on-screen instructions to interviewers, (2) editorial descriptions of specific words or phrases used, such as [phone number], and (3) explanations to the reader. Words in italics are not read out to the respondents. The bold headings (such as 'Introduction' below) are for the reader's convenience and were not read out by the interviewers.

Researchers interested in using these questions in other studies are urged to contact the research team through the Australian Research Centre in Sex, Health and Society in Melbourne for the full questionnaire.

Introduction

Hello, is this [phone number]? My name is [name]. I'm calling on behalf of a group of Australian universities. We are conducting the Australian Study of Women's [Men's] Health and

Relationships. We want to speak to a wide range of people across Australia so we're ringing computer-generated numbers in this area. [Did you receive our letter saying we would be calling your home? The letter said that we are conducting the Australian Study of Health and Relationships.]

I can explain the study to you now or I can send you a letter describing the study to any address you nominate, or I could fax or email you a copy of the letter.

This is an important study of the sexual health behaviour and attitudes of the Australian population. There is no reliable Australian information on many areas of relationships and sexual health, especially as it relates to people's everyday lives. We are interviewing people chosen at random in households across Australia.

Your household is one of those chosen to take part in this study. Of course, your participation is voluntary. All answers to questions are strictly confidential and the questions are designed so that responses are either numbers or 'yes' or 'no'.

We would very much appreciate your household's participation.

Firstly, can you tell me how many women [men] aged between 16 and 59 live in your household? It is important that I choose one person at random.

[*If parent doubtful about interview of child aged 16–18 and letter not received, send letter.*]

The computer has chosen [*person*] as the one I should speak to from your household.

Demographics

I need to ask what year you were born in. [*Prompt*: It's important we know your year of birth so we can compare responses of people of different ages. *Prompt with five-year age ranges if needed.*]

Now, to ensure we have a cross-section of people in our survey, we ask a few brief general questions about you.

Which country were you born in?

Are you of Aboriginal or Torres Strait Islander origin?
Yes / No
Aboriginal / Torres Strait Islander / Both

What year did you first arrive in Australia?

What language do you usually speak at home? [*Prompt:* By home we mean where you live.]

What is the postcode of the place you live in?
What is the name of the suburb or town? And the state?

Does anyone else beside you live in your household?

Please answer yes or no to each of the following people.
Husband or partner [*includes female partner*]?
Any children? [*Children are defined as under 16 years of age. Resident children include children under 16 who live there at least half the time.*]
How many children under five?
How many children aged five to fifteen?
Parents or parents-in-law?
Any other family members or relatives, including children 16 and over?

Anybody else?

And how many people is that all together?

In terms of legal marital status, are you—
   Never married [Includes de facto relationships if never married]
   Widowed
   Divorced
   Separated but not divorced
   Married

How old were you when you first got married?
How many times have you been married?

What is the highest educational qualification you have completed? [*Enter only one code; prompt if necessary.*]
   1   No formal schooling
   2   Primary school only
   3   Lower secondary school / School certificate / Intermediate Certificate
   4   Technical or trade certificate
   5   Higher secondary school / HSC / VCE / Leaving Certificate
   6   College certificate or diploma
   7   Undergraduate university degree
   8   Postgraduate university degree

Which of the following best describes your work status now?
You can pick more than one. [*Read out list 1–7.*]
1 Employed full-time
2 Employed part-time
3 Home duties [*Only applies if not in any other category.*]
4 Unemployed
5 Student
6 Permanently ill or unable to work
7 Retired

What is your usual job? [*Probe for enough information to allow correct allocation of ASCO codes. For unemployed, use work that respondent has done or is looking for. For retired, use last employment.*]

Sexual identity, attraction and experience

Now we would like to ask some questions about your sexual feelings and experiences. I'm now going to read out three categories and I want you to tell me the number that best describes you.

Do you think of yourself as—
1 Heterosexual or straight
2 Homosexual or lesbian [gay]
3 Bisexual
4 Queer
5 Not sure / Undecided
6 Something else / Other

Which of these six statements best describes you? I will read them out and ask you to please just give me the number. [*Order reversed for men's questionnaire.*]
1 I have felt sexually attracted only to males, never to females
2 ... more often to males, and at least once to a female
3 ... about equally often to males and to females
4 ... more often to females, and at least once to a male
5 ... only to females, never to males
6 I have never felt sexually attracted to anyone at all

In the next question when we say 'sexual experience' we mean any kind of contact with another person that you felt was sexual. It could be kissing or touching, or intercourse, or any other form of sex.

Which of these statements best describes you? Again I will read out the list and you tell me the number. [*Order reversed for men's questionnaire.*]

1 I have had sexual experiences only with males, never with females
2 ... more often with males, and at least once with a female
3 ... equally often with males and with females
4 ... more often with females, and at least once with a male
5 ... only with females, never with males
6 I have never had any sexual experience with anyone at all

Have you ever had vaginal intercourse?

First sexual experience

The next questions are about your first sexual experiences.

How old were you when you first had vaginal intercourse? [*If respondent asks about sexual contact with adults as a child:* You don't need to count anything that happened when you were very young.]

How old was your partner? [*Prompt with age ranges if needed.*]

How long had you known your partner before you had sex for the first time? [*Prompt:* 'Known' counts from when you first met in person.]

1 Less than 24 hours
2 More than a day but less than a week
3 More than a week, less than a month
4 More than a month, less than a year
5 A year or more

What was your relationship to your partner? [*If response is 'friend', probe to ascertain whether 'steady' or 'casual'.*]

1 Husband [wife]—you were married to him
2 Fiancé—you were engaged to him
3 Living together but not married
4 Steady partner [*include boyfriend*]
5 Casual partner [*include friend, workmate etc.*]
6 Sex worker

What contraception or precautions did you or your partner use that first time, if any?

1 Condom
2 Other contraception (e.g. the pill)
3 He [I] withdrew
4 Made sure it was safe period
5 No precautions

How old were you when you first had oral sex with a male? That's with his penis in your mouth, or his mouth on your vaginal area. [*If respondent asks about sexual contact with adults as a child:* You don't need to count anything that happened when you were very young.]

How old were you when you first had sex with a female? [*Let respondent use her own definition of 'had sex'. If she asks:* Not counting children's sex play. *If respondent asks about sexual contact with adults as a child:* You don't need to count anything that happened when you were very young.]
[*Prompt with age ranges if needed.*]

How long had you known your partner before you had sex for the first time? [*Prompt:* 'Known' counts from when you first met in person.]

1 Less than 24 hours
2 More than a day but less than a week
3 More than a week, less than a month
4 More than a month, less than a year
5 A year or more

What was your relationship to your partner? [*If response is 'friend', probe to ascertain whether 'steady' or 'casual'.*]

1 Living together
2 Steady partner [*include girlfriend*]
3 Casual partner [*include friend, workmate etc.*]
4 Sex worker

Number of sexual partners

The following questions are about your sexual activity with men.

In your whole life, how many men have you had vaginal or anal intercourse with? That's the man's penis in your vagina or his penis in your anus. Please include your current partner, if you have one. [*If respondent asks whether sex work is included:* Yes, we ask more about that later. *If respondent asks about sexual contact with adults as a child:* You don't need to count anything that happened when you were very young.]

[*If respondent cannot give number:* Would it be—
  1 6 to 10
  2 11 to 20
  3 21 to 30
  4 31 to 40
  5 41 to 50
  6 51 to 100
  7 101 to 500
  8 More than 500?]
[*If respondent says she has never had anal intercourse, enter code so that this is not asked later.*]

Are there any [more] men that you had oral sex with? That's the man's penis in your mouth, or his mouth on your vaginal area. Men that you didn't have vaginal or anal sex with. [*If respondent asks about sexual contact with adults as a child:* You don't need to count anything that happened when you were very young.]
How many?

Are there any [more] men that you had some form of sexual contact with that involved stimulating the penis or vaginal area? Men that you didn't have vaginal or oral sex with.
How many?
[*Similar questions were asked about vaginal or anal intercourse, oral and manual sex and condom use in the last five years and last 12 months.*]

Have you ever used condoms to have sex with a man?

Have you used condoms in the last 12 months to have sex with a man?

Have you used condoms in the last six months to have sex with a man?

Regular male partner(s)

Do you currently have a regular male sexual partner or partners? Someone you have an ongoing sexual relationship with? [*'Ongoing' means she expects the relationship to continue and to have sex with the partner again. If married and reported a partner earlier but says no here, query. May be married but living with a woman, or doesn't have sex with husband any more, but more likely doesn't realise 'sexual partner' applies to her husband.*]

Is there more than one?

Do you live with your regular partner?

How many current regular male partners do you have?

Do you live with one of these partners?

The next questions are about your regular partner. [*If she has more than one regular partner:* the regular partner you live with. *If she has non-live-in regular partners but no live-in partner:* the partner you most recently had sex with.]
How long have you been in this relationship, including any time before you were living together? [*If respondent unsure when it started:* Count from when you felt it became a regular relationship. Many people count from when they first had sex.]
__ months
Less than one year
More than one year but less than two years
More than two years but less than five years
More than five but less than 10 years
More than 10 but less than 20 years
More than 20 years

How long had you known your partner before you had sex for the first time? [*Prompt:* 'Known' counts from when you first met in person. *Respondent to use own definition of 'sex'.*]
1   Less than 24 hours
2   More than a day but less than a week
3   More than a week, less than a month
4   More than a month, less than a year
5   A year or more

How old is he?

In this relationship, do you expect that your partner would have sex only with you?

In this relationship, do you expect that you would have sex only with him?

Have you discussed these expectations with him?
Yes / No / Partly / Not sure

And have you both explicitly agreed about this?
Yes / No / Not sure

In this relationship, is any kind of contraception being used?
Yes / No / Not sure / Don't know

What form of contraception is being used? [*Ignore occasional failure to use methods.*]

1 Contraceptive pill
2 IUD
3 Depo-Provera injection
4 Implant
5 Partner has had a vasectomy
6 I have had a tubal ligation or hysterectomy
7 Condom
8 Safe period method / Natural Family Planning (rhythm method, Billings method, symptothermal, periodic abstinence)
9 Withdrawal (coitus interruptus, pulling out)
10 Douching (washing)
11 Diaphragm or cervical cap [*Prompt for foam/jelly use.*]
12 Spermicidal foam or jelly
13 Female condom
14 Other non-prescribed

Do you use that every time; or another type or method as well? [*Up to three methods recorded.*]

Can you tell me why you are not using contraception? [*Pause and allocate response to category if possible. Prompt if necessary:* Is it because you don't have intercourse, you want a baby, you are infertile, or do you have some reason you prefer not to?]

1 Not having intercourse
2 Want a baby
3 Pregnant now
4 Feeding now
5 Use safe period (periodic abstinence, rhythm method, Billings method)
6 He withdraws (pulls out)
7 Partner is infertile or subfertile
8 I am infertile
9 Have been sterilised (tubal ligation)
10 Partner has had a vasectomy
11 I have had a hysterectomy
12 I am past menopause
13 Don't care / Don't worry / Forget / Stupid / Never got pregnant
14 Don't know what to do / Don't know about methods
15 Religious objection
16 Leave it to chance / fate / God, when to have babies
17 Believe it unnatural or unhealthy
18 I experienced side effects or contraindications

19 Would like to but can't / Partner or parent doesn't allow / No access / No confidential service

20 Use method [*Go back to use of contraception question.*]

How many times in the past four weeks have you had sex with your partner? Even if this wasn't typical for you. Not just intercourse, but including other forms of sex. [*Number of times means number of sessions, not number of acts, i.e. a session of oral + intercourse + manual = one session. If they stopped for dinner or sleep and continued, that's two sessions.*]

Thinking now about your relationship with this partner. How physically pleasurable do you find sex with this partner to be? Is it—

1 Extremely pleasurable
2 Very pleasurable
3 Moderately pleasurable
4 Slightly pleasurable
5 Not at all pleasurable

How emotionally satisfying do you find your relationship with this partner to be? Is it—

1 Extremely satisfying
2 Very satisfying
3 Moderately satisfying
4 Slightly satisfying
5 Not at all satisfying

This next section is about the man you most recently had sex with. [*Repeated for second most recent and third most recent partner if applicable.*]

I am now going to ask about sex with the man that you most recently had sex with.

When was the last time you had sex with this man? By 'sex' we mean any kind of contact with another person that you felt was sexual, not just intercourse.

__ days / weeks / months ago

What was your relationship to him? [*Wait and prompt if necessary. If sex work, code response as 5, other.*]

1 Live-in partner
2 Regular partner, but not living together
3 Occasional partner
4 Casual partner or one-night stand
5 Other

Was this regular partner the one you described before? [*Or:* Was this regular partner one of the men you described before, *and if yes:* Which one, the first or the second? *as appropriate.*]
   1   Yes, the one I do not live with
   2   No, this is another regular partner I have not described
   3   Yes, the first regular partner
   4   Yes, the second regular partner

How old was he? [*Prompt with age categories if needed.*]

How long had you known him before you had sex for the first time? [*Prompt:* Known counts from when you first met in person.]
   1   Less than 24 hours
   2   More than a day but less than a week
   3   More than a week, less than a month
   4   More than a month, less than a year
   5   A year or more

How long ago was the first time you had sex with him?
   __ days / weeks / months / years ago

Did you use any contraception?
   Yes / No / Not sure / Don't know

What form of contraception did you use? [*Response options as for question on current contraceptive use above.*]

Did you use [only that *or* that every time *based on previous responses*], or another type or method as well?

Can you tell me why you did not use contraception? [*Response options and prompt as above.*]

The last time you had sex, did he put his penis into your vagina?

Was a condom used?

Was the condom put on before his penis touched your vagina?

Did he ejaculate inside you? [*If respondent states 'Yes', clarify whether ejaculation occurred in the condom.*]
   No / Yes, in the condom / Yes, not in the condom / Not sure

The last time you had sex, did he put his penis into your anus?

Was a condom used when you did this?

Was the condom put on before his penis touched your anus?

Did he ejaculate inside your rectum? [*If respondent states 'Yes', clarify whether ejaculation occurred in the condom.*]

No / Yes, in the condom / Yes, not in the condom / Not sure

The last time you had sex, did you have oral sex with your mouth on his penis?

Did you have oral sex with his mouth on your vaginal area?

Did you stimulate his penis with your hand?

Did he stimulate your clitoris or vaginal area with his hand?

And the last time you had sex with him, did you have an orgasm?

[*Sexual practices at last sexual encounter for male respondents with male partners included receptive and insertive anal intercourse. For women with female partners, only oral and manual sex were recorded.*]

In the past twelve months have you had sex with any man [person / people] other than the one [ones] you have already [just] told me about?

Last six months safe and unsafe sex with men

The following questions are about your regular male live-in partner. [*Questions repeated as appropriate for regular non-live-in partner(s).*]

During the past six months, how often did you have vaginal intercourse with your regular partner [who you live with] where he ejaculated inside you? Was that never, occasionally or often?

When you did this, how often was a condom used?
Never / Occasionally / Often

During the past six months, how often did you have vaginal intercourse with him where he withdrew before ejaculating? Was that never, occasionally or often?

When you did this, how often was a condom used? Was that never, occasionally or often?

During the past six months, how often did you have anal intercourse with him where he ejaculated inside you? Was that never, occasionally or often?

When you did this, how often was a condom used? Was that never, occasionally or often?

During past six months, how often did you have anal intercourse with your regular partner where he withdrew before ejaculating? Was that never, occasionally or often?

When you did this, how often was a condom used? Was that never, occasionally or often?

During the last six months, how often have you had oral sex with your partner's penis in your mouth? Was that never, occasionally or often?

When you did this, how often did he ejaculate in your mouth? Was that never, occasionally or often?

During the last six months, how often have you had oral sex with your partner's mouth on your vaginal area? Was that never, occasionally or often?

In the past six months, how many men [other than your regular partner] have you had sex with?

Did you have sex on more than one occasion?

During the past six months, how often did you have vaginal intercourse with a non-regular partner[s] where he [they] ejaculated inside you? Was that never, occasionally or often?

When you did this, how often was a condom used? Was that never, occasionally or often?

During the past six months, how often did you have vaginal intercourse with a non-regular partner[s] where he [they] withdrew before ejaculating? Was that never, occasionally or often?

When you did this, how often was a condom used? Was that never, occasionally or often?

During the past six months, how often did you have anal intercourse with a non-regular partner[s] where he [they] ejaculated inside you? Was that never, occasionally or often?

When you did this, how often was a condom used? Was that never, occasionally or often?

During the past six months, how often did you have anal intercourse with a non-regular partner[s] where he [they] withdrew before ejaculating? Was that never, occasionally or often?

When you did this, how often was a condom used? Was that never, occasionally or often?

During the last six months, how often have you had oral sex with a non-regular partner's penis in your mouth? Was that never, occasionally or often?

When you did this, how often did he [they] ejaculate in your mouth? Was that never, occasionally or often?

During the last six months, how often have you had oral sex with his [their] mouth[s] on your vaginal area? Was that never, occasionally or often?

Sex with women

Number of partners

The following questions are about your sexual activity with women.

[*Check previous response by stating:*] You said earlier that you have had no sexual contact with women. [*Wait for confirmation. If respondent has had sexual contact with women, continue with questions about sexual activity with women.*]

[*If respondent has stated previously that she has had sexual contact with women:* Now some questions about your sexual activity with women.]

In your whole life, how many women have you had oral sex with? That's your mouth on her vaginal area or her mouth on your vaginal area. Please include your current partner, if you have one. [*If respondent asks whether sex work is included, say:* Yes, we ask more about that later. *If she asks about sexual contact with adults as a child, say:* You don't need to count anything that happened when you were very young.]

[*If respondent cannot give number:* Would it be—

1   6 to 10
2   11 to 20
3   21 to 30
4   31 to 40
5   41 to 50
6   51 to 100
7   101 to 500
8   More than 500?]

Are there any [more] women that you had some form of sexual contact with that involved touching the vaginal area? [Women that you didn't have oral sex with.]

How many? [*Prompt with categories if needed.*]

[*Previous questions repeated for partners in the last five years and last 12 months.*]

Regular female partner(s)

The following questions are about your regular female partner[s].

Do you currently have a regular female sexual partner or partners? Someone you have an ongoing sexual relationship with. [*Ongoing means she expects the relationship to continue and to have sex with the partner again.*]

Is there more than one?

Do you live with her?

How many current regular female partners do you have?

Do you live with one of these partners?

The next questions are about the regular female partner you live with.

[*Questions repeated or replaced as appropriate with questions about female partner(s) respondent does not live with, starting with the one she most recently had sex with.*]

Last six months safe and unsafe sex with women

During the last six months, how often have you had oral sex with your partner's mouth on your genital area? Was that never, occasionally or often?

During the last six months, how often have you had oral sex with your mouth on your partner's vaginal area? Was that never, occasionally or often?

In the past six months, how many women have you had sex with [other than your regular partner(s)]?

Did you have sex on more than one occasion?

During the last six months, how often have you had oral sex with your partner's [partners'] mouth[s] on your vaginal area? Was that never, occasionally or often?

During the last six months, how often have you had oral sex with your mouth on your partner's [partners'] vaginal area[s]? Was that never, occasionally or often?

Masturbation and esoteric practices

The next section is about things that some people do to add to sexual stimulation. If you have not heard of any of the things I read out, just tell me.

In the last twelve months, have you ever masturbated alone? [*Prompt if necessary:* stimulated yourself.]

Yes / No / Not sure / Can't remember

In the last four weeks how many times have you masturbated alone? [*Orgasm is not required for activity to qualify as masturbation.*]

In the last twelve months, have you had phone sex or called a telephone sex line?

In the last twelve months, have you gone to a sex site on the Internet on purpose? [*This includes both looking at pictures and chat rooms.*]

In the last twelve months, have you met a sexual partner through an Internet chat room?

In the last twelve months, have you watched an X-rated video or film? [*X is classified as 'non-violent erotica', from sex shops or mail order in NSW. R-rated does not count.*]

In the last twelve months, have you used a sex toy such as a vibrator or dildo? [*Includes any other toys such as butt plugs, ben-wa balls etc., but not feathers, canes, massage oil etc.*]

[*From here on, if respondent doesn't understand questions or expresses discomfort, skip to next section.*]

In the last twelve months, have you been involved in role playing or dressing up? [*Includes playing games like 'naughty schoolgirl', 'captain and cabin boy' etc., or dressing up in fetish gear or, for men, women's clothing.*]

In the last twelve months, have you been involved in B&D or S&M? That's bondage and discipline, sado-masochism, or dominance and submission.

And in the last twelve months, have you been involved in group sex?

And in the last twelve months, have you used your fingers to stimulate a partner's anus, or had a partner do that to you?

And have you been involved in fisting? [*Do not explain. Includes both receptive and insertive, vaginal and rectal fisting, if respondent asks which.*]

Oral–anal contact or rimming?

Sexual forcing

The next section is about sexual situations that both women and men have encountered. We understand that sometimes these are difficult issues to discuss.

Have you ever had a sexual experience with a man or a woman when you didn't want to because you were too drunk or high at the time?
   Yes / No / Don't know / Not sure

Have you ever been forced or frightened by a man or a woman into doing something sexually that you did not want to do?
   Yes / No / Don't know / Not sure

How many times has this happened to you?
   __ times / Too often to count

How old were you at the time [when it started *or* the first time]?

Did you talk to someone else about it or seek help?
Who did you talk to?
   1   Sibling
   2   Parent
   3   Friend
   4   Rape crisis centre
   5   Hospital
   6   Police
   7   Teacher
   8   Clergy
   9   Counsellor, psychologist, etc.
   10   Doctor or nurse
   11   Magazines, newspapers, radio
   12   Spouse or partner
   13   Other relative

[*At interviewer's discretion*] If you would like I can give you a phone number of someone to talk to [more] about this. The number is [*read out appropriate number from sheet*].
   1   Respondent accepted number
   2   Respondent did not want number
   3   Interviewer did not offer

Sexual difficulties

The next questions are about your sexual life now.

During the last year has there been a period of one month or more when you lacked interest in having sex?

[If yes, the following question is asked for all the sexual difficulties mentioned.] And did that last—
1 At least one month but less than three months
2 At least three months but less than six months
3 Six months or more

Has there been a period of one month or more when you were unable to come to orgasm (a climax)?

Has there been a period of one month or more when you came to orgasm (a climax) too quickly?

Has there been a period of one month or more when you experienced physical pain during intercourse?

Has there been a period of one month or more when you did not find sex pleasurable?

Has there been a period of one month or more when you felt anxious about your ability to perform sexually?

[Has there been a period of one month or more when you had trouble keeping an erection when you wanted to?]

[Have you ever used any treatment to help with erections? For example, injections or tablets like Viagra.]

[Have you used any of these treatments in the last twelve months?]

Has there been a period of one month or more when you had trouble with vaginal dryness?

During sex do you worry whether your body looks unattractive?

Ideally, how often would you like to have sex? *[Pause and read out list with numbers.]*
1 More than once a day
2 Daily
3 Five to six times a week
4 Three to four times a week
5 Two to three times a week
6 Once a week
7 Once every two weeks
8 Once every three weeks
9 Monthly
10 Less than monthly
11 Every six months
12 Annually
13 Never

Men's difficulties with condoms

Now I'd like to ask you about condoms.

Over your lifetime how many times has a condom actually broken when having sex with another person?

In the last twelve months how many condoms have you used?
1   One
2   Two to five
3   Six to 10
4   11 to 50
5   51 to 100
6   More than 100
7   None

In the last twelve months, how often have you experienced the following difficulties with condoms? [*All answers must refer to the last twelve months.*]

The condom was broken during entry or during intercourse.
1   Never
2   Once
3   Two to five times
4   More than five times

The condom was discovered to be broken on withdrawal or taking it off.

In the last twelve months, how often has the condom slipped off during intercourse or during withdrawal?

Do you usually use extra lubricant?
[*If yes:*] What type of lubricant do you usually use? [Can you say what brand?]
1   None
2   Saliva/spit
3   Soap
4   Water-based
5   Oil-based
[*Enter brand or other type.*]

Fertility

[Section skipped if respondent has never had vaginal intercourse.]

The following questions are about contraception and pregnancy.

[*If respondent has not already been asked about contraception.*] Now I would like to ask you about contraception. [*Same questions as above on contraceptive use and reasons for non-use.*]

Have you ever used emergency contraception or the morning-after pill?
    Yes / No / Don't know what it is

How many times have you used it?

Have you ever been pregnant?
    Yes / No / Don't know

How old were you when you first became pregnant?
    __ years / Can't remember

How many children have you had? [*If she asks, this means live births, not the ones now with her.*]

Have you ever had a miscarriage? Can you please tell me how many?

Have you ever had a stillbirth? Can you please tell me how many?

Have you ever had a termination of pregnancy (i.e. an abortion)? Can you please tell me how many?

Have you ever had a child that was given up for adoption? Can you please tell me how many children?

Have you ever experienced difficulties trying to get pregnant?

Have you been treated to help you get pregnant?

Sex work

Have you ever been paid money for sex, including oral sex or manual stimulation? [*If respondent has done sex work but did not receive the money herself, code as yes.*]
    Yes / No

In your lifetime, how many men have paid money for sex with you?

How old were you the first time a man paid money for sex with you?

Did you include men who paid you when I asked you about what you usually did with casual partners in the last six months?

Of the men who have paid you, how many were outside Australia?

What country was that? [What was the main country where this occurred?]

Has a man paid money for sex with you in the last twelve months?

How many times have men paid for sex with you in the last twelve months? [*Type in number of clients, or numbers of visits if she has regular client(s).*]

What year was the last time a man paid you for sex?

In the last twelve months, how did you meet men who paid you for sex? Please tell me yes or no for each one.
    On the street?
    In a brothel, i.e. with a manager? [Includes heterosexual saunas and swingers clubs where women are paid by the house]
    In a house or flat with a small group of women?
    Escort agency?
    Massage parlour?
    Privately or informally? [Includes Internet or classified ad, if she does not work in above venues]
    Other [Includes bar girls and other arrangements overseas]

Do you usually work—
    1 Alone
    2 With a minder/sitter/partner
    3 With one other worker
    4 With several other sex workers

Thinking about the last time you were paid for sex, was this the last casual encounter you told me about earlier?
    Yes / No / Don't remember

The next few questions are about the last time a man paid you for sex, even if this was different from usual for you.

When was the last time a man paid you for sex?
    __ days / __ weeks / __ months

How old do you think he was?
1 Under 18 years
2 18 to 24 years
3 25 to 34 years
4 35 to 44 years
5 45 to 54 years
6 55 to 64 years
7 Over 65 years
8 Don't know

The last time a man paid you for sex, did he put his penis in your vagina?
Yes / No / Don't remember

Was a condom used?

Was the condom put on before the man's penis touched your vagina?

Did he ejaculate inside you?
Yes / No / Yes, in the condom / Don't remember

The last time a man paid you for sex, did he put his penis in your anus?

Was a condom used when he did this?

Was the condom put on before his penis touched your anus?

Did he ejaculate inside you?
Yes / No / Yes, in the condom / Don't remember

The last time a man paid you for sex, did you have oral sex with his penis in your mouth?

Did he ejaculate in your mouth?

Did you have oral sex with his mouth on your vaginal area?

Did you stimulate his penis with your hand?

Did he stimulate your vaginal area with his hand?

The last time a man paid you for sex, did you engage in B&D or S&M?

Have you ever been paid for sex with a woman?

Were you paid by a man or men, or by the woman?
1 By a man or men
2 By the woman
3 Both at different times

Have you ever paid money for sex, including oral sex or manual stimulation?

Have you ever paid for sex with a man? [*If she has visited a sex worker and someone else paid, code as yes.*]

How old were you the first time you paid for sex with a man?
__ years / Don't remember

In your lifetime, how many men have you paid money to for sex?

Was that in Australia? [Of those, how many were outside Australia?]

What country was that? [What was the main country where this occurred?]

Have you ever paid money for sex with a woman?

[*Questions were also asked about men's experience of paying for sex with women and with men, and about men being paid for sex with women and with men.*]

[*Asked of men:* How much did you pay, the last time you paid a woman [man] for sex?]

General health

In general, would you say your health is—[*read out options 1 to 5*]
  1 Excellent
  2 Very good
  3 Good
  4 Fair
  5 Poor
  8 Don't know

In the past four weeks, about how often did you feel nervous? All of the time, most of the time, some of the time, a little of the time or none of the time?

In the past four weeks, about how often did you feel so sad that nothing could cheer you up? [*Read scale if necessary.*]

In the past four weeks, about how often did you feel restless or fidgety?

In the past four weeks, about how often did you feel hopeless?

In the past four weeks, about how often did you feel that everything was an effort?

In the past four weeks, about how often did you feel worthless?

Do you smoke cigarettes, cigars, pipes or any other tobacco products?

Would that be—[read out scale]
1 Daily
2 At least weekly
3 Less often than weekly

Over your lifetime, would you have smoked at least 100 cigarettes or a similar amount of tobacco?

For how many years did you smoke? [If respondent has stopped and started, add the smoking periods together.]

When you smoked, how many cigarettes did you smoke a day, on average? [If respondent gives range, use middle value.]

For how many years have you smoked? [If respondent has stopped and started, add the smoking periods together.]

On average, how many cigarettes do you smoke a day? [If respondent gives range, use middle value.]

How often do you have an alcoholic drink of any kind? [If respondent gives range, use middle value.]
1 Every day
2 Six days a week
3 Five days a week
4 Four days a week
5 Three days a week
6 Two days a week
7 One day a week
8 Fortnightly or less
9 Monthly or less
10 Do not drink alcohol

On a day that you have alcoholic drinks, how many drinks do you usually have? [If respondent asks: A drink is a glass of wine or beer, or a nip of spirits. If respondent gives range, use middle value.]

Are you currently taking any medication for high blood pressure or a heart condition?

Have you ever been told by a doctor or nurse that you have diabetes or high blood sugar?
No / Yes, diabetes / Yes, high blood sugar / Don't know

Were you pregnant when you were first you had diabetes [high blood sugar]?

Have you ever had diabetes [high blood sugar] apart from when you were pregnant?

How old were you when you were first told you had diabetes [high blood sugar]?

[*Asked of men:* Have you been circumcised? [*Prompt:* Has the loose skin at the tip of your penis been removed?]]

Do you have a condition or disability that hinders your mobility?

In the last twelve months, has that condition affected you for a period of at least one month?

Sexual health and sexually transmissible infections

The following questions are about sexual health. Not all the questions are about sexually transmissible diseases.

Have you ever had any of the following? I will read out a list, and ask you to say yes or no to each one.
    Pubic lice or crabs?
    Genital warts? [*Includes anal warts if she asks.*]
    Wart virus (HPV) indication on a Pap smear?
    Chlamydia?
    Genital herpes?
    Syphilis?
    Gonorrhoea?
    [Non-specific urethritis or NSU?]
    Pelvic inflammatory disease (PID)?
    Bacterial vaginosis or gardnerella?
    Trichomoniasis or 'trike'?
    Vaginal [penile] candida or thrush?
    Hepatitis A?
    Hepatitis B?
    Hepatitis C?

[*For each condition respondent has had, the following questions are asked.*]

Have you had it [them] [an attack] in the past twelve months? [*For hepatitis A, B or C:* Was this a new infection acquired in the past twelve months?]

Where did you go for treatment for it [them]? [*If more than one place, record the first place she went in the most recent occurrence. Clarify what type of clinic if respondent just says 'clinic'.*]

1 Usual GP
2 New GP
3 24-hour clinic
4 Sexual health clinic [*STD clinic or clap clinic*]
5 Public hospital or outpatients
6 Private hospital
7 Family planning clinic
8 Alternative health professional
9 Chemist
10 Friend
11 Self-treatment
12 No treatment

Sexual attitudes

I'm now going to read a number of statements and I'd like you to tell me whether you strongly agree, agree, neither agree nor disagree, disagree or strongly disagree.

Films these days are too sexually explicit.

Sex before marriage is acceptable.

If two people had oral sex, but not intercourse, you would still consider that they had had sex together.

An active sex life is important for your sense of wellbeing.

Abortion is always wrong.

Having an affair when in a committed relationship is always wrong.

Sex tends to get better the longer you know someone.

Sex between two adult women is always wrong.

Sex between two adult men is always wrong.

Knowledge about sexually transmissible infections and blood-borne virus infections

Not many more questions to go. The following statements are about sexually transmitted diseases and hepatitis. Please answer true or false for each.

Chlamydia affects only women.

Chlamydia can lead to infertility in women.

Hepatitis C has no long-term effects on your health.

Once a person has caught genital herpes, they will always have the virus.

People who have injected drugs are at risk for hepatitis C.

Hepatitis C can be transmitted by tattooing and body piercing.

Hepatitis B can be transmitted sexually.

Gonorrhoea can be transmitted through oral sex.

Genital warts can only be spread by intercourse.

Cold sores and genital herpes can be caused by the same virus.

We now have some questions about infections that may be transmitted by blood.

As you may know, there is a blood test that tells you whether or not you have HIV, the virus that causes AIDS. Have you ever had a blood test for HIV?
  Yes / No / Don't know / Not sure

When did you have the last test?

Did your most recent test show that you— [*Only read out codes 1 and 2.*]
  1   Have the virus (HIV positive)
  2   Do not have the virus (HIV negative)
  3   Waiting for the results
  4   Did not get the results

Do you personally know, or have you personally known, someone who has AIDS or is HIV-positive?
  Yes / Yes, knew someone in the past / No / Don't know / Not sure

Have you ever injected (self-injected) any drugs, apart from prescribed drugs? [*Includes respondent being injected by someone else. Includes heroin, speed, cocaine, ecstasy, steroids or any recreational drugs.*]

In the last twelve months, have you injected any drugs, apart from prescribed drugs? [*Includes heroin, speed, cocaine, ecstasy, steroids or any recreational drugs.*]

I'm going to read out some drugs. Please tell me for each one (yes or no) whether you have injected it in the last twelve months.

Heroin? [*smack, hammer, 'H', horse*]
Methadone?
Other opiates? [*includes morphine, pethidine*]
Amphetamines? [*speed, go, uppers, MDA*]
Cocaine? [*coke, flake, snow; also includes crack*]
LSD or other hallucinogens? [*acid, trips, tabs, mushrooms, mescalin*]
Ecstasy? [*'E', eckie, vitamin e, MDMA*]
Benzodiazepines? [*benzos, tranqs, moggos, ro-ies, vees*)
Steroids?
Other drugs?

Where do you usually get needles and syringes from?
1   Chemist
2   Needle and syringe program
3   Friends
4   Hospital or doctor

Have you ever used a needle after someone else had already used it?
Yes / No / Don't know / Not sure

How long ago was the last time?
1   Less than one month ago
2   Between one and twelve months ago
3   Between one and five years ago
4   More than five years ago

In the last one month, when you used a needle that had already been used by someone else, did you always clean the needle and syringe using bleach?

Have you ever shared a filter, water, spoon, foil, or equipment such as a tourniquet with another drug user?

How long ago was the last time?
1   Less than one month ago
2   Between one and twelve months ago
3   Between one and five years ago
4   More than five years ago

Have you ever been vaccinated against hepatitis A?

Have you ever been vaccinated against hepatitis B?

Have you ever been tattooed?

Were any of your tattoos done in the last twelve months?

Where did you go to have the last tattoo done? [*Prompt if necessary.*]
  1 At tattoo parlour / professional
  2 At home / friend's
  3 In prison
  4 Overseas

Including earrings, have you had any body piercings in the last twelve months?

At what place was it done? [*Prompt if necessary.*]
  1 At a parlour / professional
  2 Chemist / beauty salon / hairdresser
  3 At home / friend's
  4 In prison
  5 Overseas

Have you ever been detained in a prison or a juvenile detention facility for more than 24 hours [in the last 15 years]?

Now, a few final questions.

Do you have a particular religion or faith?
  Yes / No ['No' means no religion]

What religion or faith do you follow?
  1   Anglican / Church of England
  2   Baptist
  3   Catholic
  4   Lutheran
  5   Oriental Christian
  6   Orthodox Christian
  7   Presbyterian and Reformed
  8   Uniting Church
  9   Other Christian
  10 Buddhist
  11 Islam / Muslim
  12 Other non-Christian

How often do you attend services or meetings? [*Prompt if necessary. If only attends at festivals (Easter, Christmas etc.), code as 3, less than monthly.*]
  1 Never
  2 Only on special occasions (weddings, funerals, christenings etc.)
  3 Less than monthly
  4 Monthly
  5 Weekly
  6 Daily

What is your approximate family income before tax and other deductions? That's the total for you, your partner and your children if they live at home. I'll read out the categories and you just give me the number. [*Read out 1–5. Clarify that the amount is before tax, super, health insurance etc. are deducted.*]

1 Under $11 000 per year
2 $11 001 to $20 000
3 $20 001 to $32 000
4 $32 001 to $52 000
5 Over $52 000
6 Only know per week
7 Only know personal income

Would it be— [*Read out list with numbers.*]

1 Under $200 per week
2 $201 to $400
3 $401 to $600
4 $601 to $1000
5 Over $1000

What is your approximate personal income before tax and other deductions? I'll read out the categories and you just give me the number. [*Clarify that the amount is before tax, super, health insurance etc. are deducted.*]

1 Under $11 000 per year
2 $11 001 to $20 000
3 $20 001 to $32 000
4 $32 001 to $52 000
5 Over $52 000
6 Only know per week

Would it be— [*Read out list with numbers.*]

1 Under $200 per week
2 $201 to $400
3 $401 to $600
4 $601 to $1000
5 Over $1000

That's the end of the study questions, but as this is the first time this type of study has been done in Australia I'd like to ask two quick questions about the questionnaire.

How embarrassing did you find the questionnaire?
1 Extremely embarrassing
2 Very embarrassing
3 Quite embarrassing
4 Slightly embarrassing
5 Not at all embarrassing

In percentage terms, how honest were you in your answers to the questionnaire?

That's it. Thank you for your help. In case you missed it, my name is [name] calling on behalf of a group of Australian Universities. If you have any concerns or questions, you are welcome to call our free phone number [phone number].

Thank you once again.

index